THE DAY I DIED

THE DAY I DIED

ONE MAN'S SUCCESSFUL BATTLE BACK FROM THE DEAD

Jay Barbree

NEW HORIZON PRESS
Far Hills, New Jersey

Library of Congress Catalog Card Number: 90-53405

Jay Barbree
  The Day I Died

ISBN: 0-88282-061-3
New Horizon Press

For

David Frank

Pat Sullivan

Debi Hall

Ed Clemons

Lee Proctor

&

Chris Bedard

THE LIFESAVERS

CONTENTS

INTRODUCTION

by Onkar S. Narula M.D.

Jay Barbree, the author of this book, is one of those rare individuals who was lucky enough to have survived sudden cardiac death. He is unique due to the fact that afterward he took charge of his life to modify his destiny. He actively participated in selecting medical facilities and deciding therapeutic options. He undertook measures to prevent a recurrence and succeeded. This autobiography deals with his predetermined destiny, survival, strength, and determination.

Sudden cardiac death, sometimes called SCD, is defined as an unexpected rapid cardiac death occurring without symptoms or with symptoms of less than one hour duration. It is the most common mode of death. In the United States alone approximately half a million people per year, or one person per minute, experience sudden cardiac death. Only 20-30 percent of the latter survive. Those who do so receive cardiopulmonary resuscitation (CPR) within a few minutes of its occurrence by someone at the scene or by a paramedic rescue squad called in time. Sudden cardiac death remains a major unresolved health problem due to a 70-80 percent mortality rate. The survivors of SCD require thorough evaluation for institution of appropriate therapeutic measures to prevent its recurrence. The challenge is to identify patients at high risk of SCD, and to institute measures to modify the risks and to devise an effective therapy.

1

Sudden cardiac death is caused by a malfunction of the electrical system of the heart. Eighty to ninety percent of SCDs are due to an abnormal rapid and erratic beating of the two lower chambers. Only a small percentage of SCDs (10-20 percent) result from a lack of heart beat and heart stoppage.

The major (80 percent) cause of SCD is coronary artery disease sometimes called CAD. In the majority (75 percent) of the cases, it leads to disturbances of the electrical system of the heart. Diseased coronary arteries clogged with cholesterol deposits may restrict or completely obstruct blood flow to the heart. A totally clogged coronary artery may lead to complete cessation of blood flow, and thus deprives the heart muscle of its oxygen supply, resulting in damage to the muscle and a heart attack. Acute damage to the heart muscle (acute myocardial infarction) is responsible for SCD in only 20 percent of cases. In the remaining 80 percent of the cases, SCD is not associated with an acute damage to the muscle. In these cases, SCD results: when, during periods of physical or emotional stress, increased demands for blood supply are not met in persons with partially clogged coronary arteries, which are unable to increase blood flow in keeping with the increased demand. Oxygen deprivation leads to electrical malfunction and an erratic, rapid heart beat and SCD. The heart muscle damaged during a heart attack is replaced by scar tissue which, when interspersed with normal muscle fibers spared from the damage, produces electrical short circuits and erratic heart beat. Therefore, some patients with an old heart attack are at risk for SCD even in the absence of oxygen deprivation to the heart muscle or a new heart attack. In a small number of cases SCD occurs despite normal coronary arteries. In these individuals, it is caused by other cardiac abnormalities.

Survivors of SCD have a 30 percent risk of recurrence within one year if left untreated or inadequately managed. Therefore, these cases merit thorough evaluation and institution of preventive, as well as curative measures.

Coronary artery disease is an extremely common and highly lethal disease. Data from the Framinham Study suggest that one in five adults may have a heart attack before reaching age sixty. This disease can be asymptomatic in its most severe form. Approximately one-third of all heart attacks go unrecognized. Unfortunately one in five heart attacks presents with Sudden Cardiac Death the first, last, and only symptom.

CAD due to a variety of predisposing risk factors causes clogging of the coronary arteries. These include elevation of cholesterol, high blood pressure, diabetes, and elevated fibrinogen levels. The role of elevated fat levels (triglycerides) is uncertain; however, current evidence suggests it to be an independent risk factor, especially in women.

The clogging of coronary arteries results from elevation of *total cholesterol,* especially of its bad component called low density lipoprotein, or from low levels of its good component called high density lipoprotein.

Since Jay was at high risk of Sudden Cardiac Death, additional preventive measures were undertaken to prevent ischemia (oxygen-starved heart muscle) induced arrhythmia. He was advised against unlimited vigorous exercise. Drugs were prescribed to reduce oxygen demand by the heart, to control blood pressure, and to limit the normal increase in heart rate associated with exercise or emotional stress. For this purpose, he was given beta-blockers and calcium-blocking drugs. In addition, he received anti-arrhythmic drug therapy to increase the threshold for occurrence and prevention of dangerous erratic rapid heart beat. For this purpose, he was given an age-old anti-arrhythmic drug called Quinidine.

He also tried to modify his behavior. However, he had no control over poor genetic factors. He could not alter his family history of coronary artery disease which had struck his father and a brother at a young age. Since he could not alter his genetics, the CAD did not regress; however, because of his behavioral and drug program it probably progressed at a slower rate.

He is to be congratulated, as he succeeded in his efforts. Although he ultimately needed surgery, it was delayed by two years. Disease progression was not only slowed, but was limited to only one vessel, requiring a single bypass. Not only did he undertake preventive measures to alter the course of disease progression, but he closely monitored its outcome to select the appropriate time for the next step, a revascularization procedure. This was important to avoid undergoing surgery too early, as bypass grafts do not last forever. An early intervention may require reoperation at a future date with the occurrence of bypass graft deterioration. On the other hand, undue delay in bypass surgery may lead to a heart attack and muscle damage.

He and his cardiologist, Dr. Rajan, undertook an appropriate course for management of survivors of SCD. He was immediately referred to a center capable of providing comprehensive evaluation and care. These investigations demonstrated that the malfunction of the electrical system of Jay's heart was secondary to CAD. During jogging, his heart muscle was deprived of adequate oxygen supply due to an increase in oxygen demand caused by strenuous exercise. This led to electrical instability and sudden death. After complete evaluation, the tests results were discussed with him. He was an active participant in the decisions and in the selection of the course charted for his medical management. He was offered a number of conventional alternatives: one was coronary artery bypass surgery, with or without implantation of an AICD device; the second was angioplasty, which entailed a higher risk due to the location of his obstruction; and the third was the use of anti-arrhythmic drugs which had the potential for major side effects.

He was given another option, which required that he undertake a strict regimen to produce either regression of CAD or delay its progression by altering the various risk factors; reduce oxygen demands of the heart with appropriate drugs and control of blood pressure; increase the threshold for occurrence of arrhythmia with anti-arrhythmic drugs; and avoid undue strenuous physical stress. He chose the latter path which permitted him to safely embark on a course to alter his prognosis and fate.

His inspiring autobiography emphasizes the need for active participation by the patient in the planning and decision making processes to choose the best therapeutic regimen suited for the individual. Each individual should get educated about his or her disease process, and should ask appropriate questions when selecting a medical facility, a physician and the medical regimen planned. Patient involvement in these processes plays a very important role in the ultimate outcome of the patient's fate.

Our goal should be identification of individuals at high risk of development of coronary artery disease and its prevention by modification of the predisposing risk factors. In truth, the occurrence of a coronary attack should be regarded as a preventive failure both on the part of the physician and the individual.

PROLOGUE

A jogger doesn't begin his run with the thought that it will end in death. I surely didn't on May 28th, 1987. Those of us on the white sands of Cocoa Beach, Florida were enjoying a typical late spring day. The temperature was in the mid-eighties, and you could feel the first wave of approaching summer. Taut sails pushed riders on fast-moving wheels along the beach, while across the brilliant blue sea a cruise ship hung like a slow-moving cloud where the ocean and sky come together.

It was good to be home. As an NBC News Correspondent, I had just returned from covering the Challenger disaster, its aftermath and the recovery.

I could feel my body settling comfortably into the run. There was no stress, no extra effort. It was something I had done many times before, and it felt as natural as a late-evening stroll.

Now I checked my watch. The run was twenty-five minutes old. Just ahead, just past home, was the finish point.

I was not aware of what was going on inside my chest. There was no pain. Only exhaustion.

The heart was entering ventricular fibrillation. The electrical seizure was causing it to beat in a rapid, unsyn-

chronized, uncoordinated fashion. It was no longer pumping blood. It seemed like a bundle of squirming worms.

My knees felt weak. My body went limp. I fell on my side with my arm resting under my head. Suddenly there was only blackness. A pure, deep blackness, absent of dreams.

The heart quivered to a stop. It refused to beat.
Jay Barbree knew nothing. He was dead.

*I*n a unit on the third floor of the Park Place Condominium, Debi Hall was busy preparing dinner, annoyed with her detective husband for leaving the police radio on. The constant 10-4s and law enforcement chatter were getting on her nerves.

She paid scant attention to the call that a man was down on the beach and the Rescue Squad was rolling, until she heard the location.

Then, she ran to the balcony, looked down and saw a lifeless body.

On her way out the door, she only stopped long enough to turn off the stove.

Her reaction was a normal one for Debi. She had been trained as an emergency medical technician to quickly react to any life-threatening situation. Her job was to take care of workers on the nation's spaceport at the Kennedy Space Center, including the astronauts.

Within seconds she was on the beach.

First, she checked for a pulse. There was none. Then she resumed CPR. She knew it was critical to keep oxygen and blood moving to the brain and other vital organs.

She completed a sequence and shouted in Barbree's ear. "Don't go to the light! Don't go to the light! You're gonna' be all right."

Her efforts were tireless. She kept the rhythm going. "Where the hell is that Rescue Squad?" she yelled.

ONE

"The Boyhood Years"

Mornings came early to the farmlands of southwest Georgia. November 26th, 1933 was no exception. It came with roosters crowing, before the sun rose above fields swirling with furrows, each fresh with frost on stubble of burnt cotton, peanut and corn stalks laying dormant, waiting for spring planting. It came with the pungent smell of home-cut bacon frying, biscuits baking, the welcome aroma of coffee perking and grits boiling in an open kettle. It came to a house that was almost naked, a forbidding and weathered structure unrelieved by any plants but the patch of dead cotton stalks clambering at a wire fence.

Will Barbree worked his toes into his shoes, rose from the bed and walked to the window, opened it, and poked his head outside. He sniffed the fresh scent of frost, and studied his fields. He heard a song floating in the air of first light, a yearning, soaring harmony through the chilly atmosphere. He could not make out the words, but it was a happy song. It ebbed back upon the dormant fields and sank away into a humming that swelled hoarsely out of throats and chests.

He turned from the window and, between beds stacked closely together in two large rooms, he steered a course outside, across the back porch, and down a well-used path to the outhouse.

His morning relief accomplished, Will Barbree returned to the back porch where a plank had been nailed to support a face pan. He poured icy water into the basin and lifted a bar of home-made soap. He splashed the cold water onto his face and scrubbed his hands, wiping them dry with a nearby towel.

He cleared his throat and went into the kitchen where an old ice box and a wood stove hugged the wall on his right, and on his left, an aged hutch held dishes, saucers, cups, bowls, and all the items needed to set the linoleum-top table in the center of the room.

"Morning, honey," he said, watching his wife, Jeannie, turn several sizzling slices of the home-cut-bacon in an iron skillet. "Is the coffee ready?"

Jeannie lifted a grey-specked pot from the cast-iron wood stove and began to pour. She was a small woman with shining eyes, but a very pregnant woman.

"Think the baby'll be here today?" Will asked.

"No," she shook her head. "Figure we've got another week, maybe more."

She turned back to her stove to conceal the worry in her face. The worry wasn't new. Anxiety had been in Jeannie Sheffield Barbree from the day she was born. She was one of seven children in a house where there was never enough to go around. And since she and Will had been married, going on twenty-two years, she had had six children of her own, two of whom were already in their graves.

Four years earlier the family had returned from living in Florida with just enough money to buy the small farm. The Depression had hit them hard, as it had everyone else, and they had to take in Will's father. He died a year later, and now her own father was in the house, sharing what little they had.

Everyone did the best they could, but the Depression kept taking its toll. Every week she would learn of some old folks or babies being carried to the cemetery, dead of starvation, and almost as often, someone they knew would disappear from the farmlands. Soon as a boy was old enough he would hop a freight, but marriage was the only escape for a girl.

Her eldest, Lois, was living in Columbus, married to a man with a good job, but her son, Larry, was not yet old enough to leave. He was only thirteen. Jean was six. Billie was almost two. They all had to be fed, and now there was another on the way.

The new baby would need milk. Her breasts had dried up, refused to nurse babies two children ago, and she didn't know where money would come from to buy "Eagle" canned milk.

She looked at Will drinking his coffee and reminded herself they would manage. They always had, she thought with a smile as she watched Billie come into the kitchen, rubbing sleep from her eyes.

The tot's tiny body was clothed in a nightgown her mother had cut and sown from a flour sack, and she placed her head on her father's knee. "Breakfast ready yet, momma?"

"It sure is for momma's big girl," Jeannie smiled. "Go get everybody up, honey, and we'll eat."

Jeannie's face brightened as she reminded herself to thank God for four, uh, soon five healthy children.

Will Barbree and his son, Larry, left the breakfast table for the fields, and the day moved through its morning like most of the others that had gone before. Jean and Billie played together until Grandpa Sheffield decided he needed to take a walk. Jean went along and Billie decided it was time to eat again—an early habit of snacking she would never overcome.

Jeannie was in the kitchen, baking more biscuits, planning the midday meal, what farmers in the area called dinner, when the first pain hit.

It seemed to be nothing. Only a pain akin to her first menstrual cramps. She ignored it and turned her attention to Billie's whining. The tot wanted dinner early and she was in no mood to take no for an answer.

Her mother tried to console her, assure her they would all have dinner shortly, but that wouldn't please the little girl.

Pain? Sharper this time. Pain she had felt many times before. Unmistakeable pain. Pains of birth.

She began to move things off the wood stove and banked the fire within the iron grates. Then she opened the oven and tried to explain to Billie she would have to wait.

"Where's Jean?" she asked. "Where's Larry? Where's Grandpa?" She walked to the front door, stared across the dirt yard toward the dirt road that ran north and south before their farm. There was no one. She and an almost two-year-old were alone.

She turned back to the kitchen, Billie pulling at her dress, still demanding something to eat when a stronger, more persistent pain hit.

No denying it this time. The contractions were coming, closer together, and she felt her water break. She was essentially alone. Only one thing to do. Go to the bed. Get in the bed and hope Grandpa and Jean would return soon.

She moved slowly and carefully to her bed, weakness sweeping her body. *Pain.* The pains of birth were coming more quickly now and she still had Billie pulling on her dress, crying for something to eat.

She reached the bed and sat down. Her legs were heavy, very heavy. Someone had filled them with sand, she thought as she lifted her left one onto the bed. It was an almost impossible job, but she made it, and she decided to rest for a while—wait until she had the strength to lift the right one.

But the baby wasn't waiting. She felt it coming into the world and there was nothing she could do about it.

Suddenly, on the bed before Billie's tear-soaked eyes a baby appeared, blue and bloody and covered with afterbirth. Jeannie reached down, lifted the baby to a dry spot on the bed, listened as the tiny boy's first cry filled the weathered wood that was the framed house.

Billie's eyes grew large and the tot stood there in total disbelief. Suddenly there were no more tears from her. Only from the baby before her, and she turned toward the door to see Jean and Grandpa Sheffield returning.

She ran to meet them, pointing back at the bed. "Baby," she cried. "Baby."

"Go to the field, Jean," the new mother said. "Go to the field and get your daddy, get Larry."

Jean was only six, but a brave six, and she ran out the door into the fields and within minutes she had found her father with a team of mules pulling out stumps, clearing new ground.

"It's the baby, Daddy," she screamed. "It's the baby."

Will stopped the team. "Go to the house and help your mother, son," he told Larry. "I'll unhitch the mules and bring them along as quickly as I can."

Larry was off in a flash, Jean close behind. With long strides across the fields, within moments they were at the house, and Larry went inside to help. His mother didn't need him. She and the baby were doing fine. What she needed was Mrs. Oscar Evans, the midwife.

Larry tore out the door and headed across the fields toward the midwife's house. Jean was close behind and Grandpa Sheffield thinking he would help, took out after them. Again, Jeannie was left alone with only a confused child. Billie decided she would go too, and in spite of her mother's pleading for her not to leave, the twenty-three-month-old toddled across the back porch and into the yard.

Her mother could no longer see her. She could not move. She could only lay there and hold onto the baby when suddenly she heard a screeching, penetrating cry from Billie. "My God," she spoke only to herself. "The hogs have got her. The hogs have got her."

It seemed like hours when it was really only minutes that she lay there, listening to Billie scream until Will reached the house with the team.

He came through the door with a sobbing Billie under his arm, and stopped before the bed.

"What happened?" his wife demanded.

"Oh, she's all right," he grinned. "She was hung up trying to crawl over the fence."

"The hogs didn't get her?"

"Nope," he smiled, putting his tiny daughter down as he began to study his new son. "It's a boy, huh?"

"A boy," Jeannie smiled.

Larry and Jean and Grandpa all returned with Mrs. Evans, and the midwife took immediate charge. You didn't easily kill a two-year-old, even in those unforgiving days, and Billie was permitted to live, to be a future companion for the new baby who would later be called Jay.

Of course, I can't remember my own birth, but I can remember when I was little more than one year old—when I was a toddler, training to make it through the day without a diaper.

My sister, Lois, and her husband Dee Miller had driven down from Columbus for a holiday visit and Dee was most proud of a Panama hat he was wearing. It was the "in" thing during Christmas 1934, but for a one-year-old who was looking for a place to take a bowel movement, the white hat was an inviting depository.

Dee had left it in the front room and while the family enjoyed dinner, I toddled into the room alone where I found that the fashionably smart hat served as a perfect chamber pot.

After my deposit was complete, only minutes passed before it was discovered and Dee demanded that I be cut up in little pieces to be used as catfish bait.

Needless to say I was never Dee Miller's favorite brother-in-law, but I wasn't through relieving myself in forbidden places.

During the great depression there were few automobiles, with even less hope of gas for their tanks. Most were pulled by horses or mules. They were called "Hoover Buggies," after the man who occupied the White House ahead of President Franklin D. Roosevelt.

My father had an old car and it was seldom we got enough gas to take a short ride, let alone make a trip to the nearby town of Blakely.

But one Saturday we got lucky. My father managed to get his hands on two gallons of gasoline and my brother Larry was excited with the knowledge he would be permitted to do the driving.

We were going to take a trip, a long trip. A fourteen-mile

trip there, and a fourteen-mile trip back from town, and everyone was so happy that even at the age of two I wanted to see this happiness last as long as possible, and something just told me that the gas would last for many more miles if I would just relieve myself in the tank. I did, and we made it about five miles from the house when the car stalled.

A fretting father and an angry brother spent most of the morning blowing the urine out of the gasoline line and clearing it from the carburetor before our journey could continue.

To this day, I have never confessed. The family is still convinced we were stranded on the road by rainwater seeping into the car's tank.

Those were not only days that saw "Hoover Buggies" as the standard mode of transportation. They were days when people traded what they had—eggs, chickens, syrup—for the things they needed.

There was no money. But a few lucky ones like my father landed jobs with President Roosevelt's WPA (Works Progress Administration).

The WPA was a government project cooked up by Roosevelt to get people out of the bread lines, to get them working again, to get a little cash in their pockets.

It was very little cash, $1.00 per day, but my father and all the WPA workers were glad to get it.

I remember how he would get up at 4:00 A.M., how my mother would fry him the one egg a day the family could afford to have, and put it inside a biscuit for a sandwich. She would pack it inside a tin syrup bucket along with anything else she could find for his lunch.

It was this egg sandwich, when I was only two or three, that gives me my earliest recollection of the good luck that would follow me through my life.

My father would return from working on the WPA—digging ditches, building roads, clearing waterways—a couple of hours after dark, about our bed time, and inside that tin syrup bucket there would always be left for me one bite of that egg sandwich.

To me, it was better than any possible treat kids enjoy

today, but it also made me feel ashamed. My sisters Billie and Jean, and brother Larry, had to go without.

Soon, I realized my good fortune was due to the fact I was the youngest, and I began to share with Billie and Jean. Larry pumped out his chest and said that, as a teenager, he was too old. It was a sharing that bonded our love more tightly, and, in later years at school, if anyone picked on any one of us, that person had us all to fight.

It was this bonding that brought us through what was to be the most traumatic event of our young lives.

I was eight years old that February day when the school bus brought Billie and me home—home to a yard filled with cars and neighbors.

We both knew something was wrong and we raced into the new house my father had built only two years before, into his room where he was lying in bed.

Several of his friends had gathered around and, as always, my father was joking, laughing with them about many memories.

Our mother took us aside and told us our daddy had come home from the fields sweating, pale white, complaining of chest pains.

My mother told us he had been wrestling with a stump in the field, trying to pry it out of the ground by himself, when he was stricken.

He was taken to the Doctor's office where there was no mention of a heart attack (the Doctor would later say he didn't want to worry him more than was necessary), and was given a shot and sent home to bed rest.

There was nothing said about keeping him quiet, and my father's friends thought they were doing the right thing, cheering him up, keeping him from worrying.

I don't know if my father knew he had had a heart attack, but I suspect he did. His brother, Remus, had died three months earlier from a heart attack, the beginning of what would later become known as the Barbree curse.

My father's father lived to be eighty, but his mother died

in her forties of heart disease, passing on early deaths through her genes to her three sons.

I wasn't old enough to grasp the significance of the moment since my father seemed his "same-old-self." He assured his friends he would be all right and they left as my mother began preparing the evening meal we called supper.

It was February, 1942. Little more than two months after the Japanese had bombed Pearl Harbor, and in spite of the war, things were better on the farm—there was more to eat.

We butchered our own hogs and with plenty of fresh milk, butter and eggs, our diet was rich in animal fats. We had no way of knowing we were eating our way into early graves.

Some people today insist our parents and forefathers were healthier than we are. They insist people of an earlier day lived longer.

The facts do not support that opinion.

What kept farmers in good health before World War II was the clean air they breathed and the hard work that burned much of the fat before it could add pounds to their bodies.

In the last century, the average person in this country died in their forties. In 1942, the average life span was in the sixties. Today, it's in the seventies and growing.

Of course, there have always been exceptions. A few people lived into their eighties and nineties in those early days—some drank, smoked, and were overweight. But, as the experts say, only ten percent of us can get away with these lifestyles. The ten percent with long-life genes.

But, because of the genes carrying heart disease that were passed on to my father from his mother, he and his brothers were in the ninety percent.

He was fifty-two, overweight, a smoker, and since it was plentiful, a big eater of meat, eggs, and milk. Even the healthy foods, the fresh garden vegetables, the peas, the beans and grains, were cooked with chunks of animal flesh, with butter saturating the biscuits and muffins.

To us, and those who had just lived through the Depression, this abundance of food was a blessing.

My father's last dinner was more of the same, a heavy meal in a body that had just suffered a heart attack—a body with a damaged heart that needed rest, as much oxygen-rich blood as it could receive through what must have been a network of severely clogged coronary arteries.

After dinner he asked for the radio to be turned up to one of his favorite programs as we all prepared for bed.

I was dozing, slipping off into sleep when I heard him begin to gasp for air.

It was an awful, struggling sound, and we all ran to his bedside, watched that friendly and understanding face twitch in pain, listened in shock as his efforts to breathe failed.

Thank God it was over in less than a minute, and I just stood there, disbelieving, as my mother screamed for my sisters Jean and Billie to run to our Uncle Louis' house for help.

There was really no need to run, there was nothing anyone could have done for my father. CPR was a procedure of the future, even pounding on a heart attack victim's chest to stimulate the heart had not been tried. We were helpless.

After things had settled down, there was stunning quiet. I walked over to my father, placed a hand on his forehead, and spoke to him. "Daddy? Daddy, can you hear me?"

Of course, there was no response, but to a boy of eight it seemed like a reasonable thing to do. It seemed like I could still talk to this man who had been so understanding, who had been my "buddy," who had worked so long and hard to take care of us.

Death to an eight-year-old is not as permanent as it is to an adult.

We buried my father and again we were faced with hard times. There was no social security in those days. Not really. The program was in its infancy and there was nowhere for a family without means to turn.

We had our farm, some hogs and chickens and a couple of milk cows, even two teams of mules to work the land, but no one to work the fields.

My brother, Larry, was in the Army, getting ready to go overseas to fight the Nazis, and my sister Jean, only fourteen, managed to get a job as a telephone operator in nearby Blakely, but my mother, my sister, Billie, and me were left on the farm.

Soon, after my mother had sold the livestock to pay the taxes on the place, we were broke.

My mother would hire out to work in the fields of other farmers for a dollar a day, and Billie would try to help. They decided I was too young, so I was sent off to spend the day with Aaron McMullen, my best friend.

My good luck was with me. It was the worst of times, but each day I was invited by Aaron's parents to eat with them and I had plenty. My poor mother and sister ate what we called "puss gravy" and biscuits.

Each week our mother would take a couple of dollars from what she had earned and buy a sack of flour and some cooking oil. From this she would make the gravy and the biscuits.

We lived like this for several months until my brother managed to get a government allotment approved from his Army pay, and we once again had the means to survive.

Then my sister Jean lied about her age, enlisted in the Women's Army Corps and managed to send us an allotment.

Again, it was the best of times, and my sister Billie and I had a chance to be kids before we were forced to grow up.

With our friend, Aaron, we would be off to the woods on summer days when birds were bullets on wings. When red-winged blackbirds would prance on tree branches, beating their wings like the devil to scare us away from their nests.

We would run over logs across the creeks, the water beneath filled with fish . . . redbreast bream around sunken logs . . . wamouth perch around the stumps. Billie would always want to stop and fish for them, but Aaron and I had other things to do—battles to be fought, bad guys to be captured.

And when our wars were won, we would be off to Howard's Mill, to the best dang swimming hole around, where we would shed our shirts, and with our overalls still on, our bare feet would kick us upward from the Mill's porch, sending our bodies soaring outward, splashing into the pond. We would come up gulping air, swimming madly. Aaron's skin brown-smooth. My own sun-red and freckled.

There were the days we'd be off to the swamp, hiding from each other as we played "Cowboys and Indians," and there was the time Aaron came running out of his hiding place, yelling he had found the biggest rattlesnake God had ever made. We found us two big sticks and ran back to the spot, and the rattlesnake was still there, all curled up, and we killed it. A thick-tailed rattler, so old his tail was missing its rattles.

And there were the nights. Nights without city lights. Nights as dark as when God created them, and we would get out of bed, go out on the front porch and lie down under the black sky. The moon was so big you could almost reach up and touch its cratered surface, and the stars were so many it seemed like the beginning of the world and we were the only people born. We would stay there until the sky grew purple, the stars dimmed, the moon set, the clouds floated into view and parted as the sun rose and sprayed new warmth.

The days passed and suddenly the family was no more. My mother remarried, my brother was back from the war, and my sisters took husbands. There was no longer a home for a sixteen-year-old boy.

There was only a few ways for a farm boy to make any ready cash in those days. He could clean manure out of barn stalls and sell the foul-smelling fertilizer to north Florida's tobacco farms, or he could wade into nearby swamps and cut cypress fence posts for sale on the town square.

My brother Larry and I had had our fill of hauling manure. We had been doing it off and on for months, and we decided to cut cypress fence posts to buy me the ticket needed to reach Kentucky where my mother lived.

I began looking for a way out. Go into the service, everyone said. I decided it was time for another Barbree to lie about his age to enter the military.

The only way I could enter the military was for my mother to sign that I was seventeen years old, and she did.

Again, good luck was with me. There were more than

250 trying to enlist in the Army and Air Force on March 2nd,
1950 in Owensboro, Kentucky, and one of my stepbrothers,
Lenord Wheatley, a Master Sergeant in the Army, spoke to
the recruiters. I was one of only three who scored high
enough to enter the Air Force. Fifty-four made it into the
Army. The rest were sent home.

After basic training in Texas, I was assigned to Scott
AFB, Illinois where I spent my off-time completing my high
school education, and watching the fighters and bombers
claw into the sky from Scott Field.

Sometimes I would walk to the end of the runway in
use and stand, gaping, as a P-51 fighter thundered over my
head, tucking up its gear and fleeing like a mighty bird into
puffy white clouds.

There was no question. I was in awe of flying machines,
and I spent much of my spare time at nearby Lebert Field in
Lebanon, Illinois, staring at the planes.

I had no money for flying lessons, but I would stand
there, watch the pilots shout "Contact!" to the mechanics,
watch as the wooden props would swing down suddenly and
catch with a stuttering cough. I loved to stand behind the
ships when the pilots revved them up for a power check. The
air blast whipped back, throwing up dust, stinking of oil and
gasoline. It flattened the grass, blew strong and heady into
my face.

Soon, I was an airport fixture. I was the pilots "go-fer." I
gladly ran their errands and helped them with their planes,
and they repaid me with local rides.

I'll never forget my first hop. The airplane was old, its
fabric a faded, splotched yellow, and the engine dripped oil.
It smelled of gasoline in flight, it shook my teeth, but I didn't
care. I loved the clanking, wheezing machine.

After a few weeks, the pilots let me handle the stick and
rudder pedals in flight, adding instructions when possible.

Then there was the day the man with the red-and-white
Stearman biplane landed at Lebert Field. I helped the pilot
with the beautiful ship, running behind the right wing and
pushing on the struts. We got the machine refueled, and I
answered all the pilot's questions, bringing him coffee and a
couple of fresh doughnuts. And while he downed the coffee,

I stood on a box, cleaning the cockpit glass, polishing the gleaming red-and-white surface here and there as the pilot watched in silence.

"Hey, kid!" he shouted. "Would you like a ride?"

My grin answered the question and minutes later we were in the air where, for the first time, I experienced aerobatics.

I'll never forget it; my introduction to that part of flight where earth and sky vanished and reappeared with startling rapidity.

It began with me staring at a vertical horizon and realizing the edge of the world now stood on its end. But not for long, as the Stearman continued on over, rolling around the inside of an invisible barrel in the air, until the ground was up and the sky was down. I had just enough time to catch my breath when the nose went down and an invisible hand pushed me gently into my seat and glued me there as the nose came up, and up. The horizon disappeared again, and the engine screamed with the dive. Then the nose was coming up, higher and higher, and the engine began to protest the pull against it. The sun flashed in my eyes, and I found myself on my back as the Stearman soared up and over in a beautiful loop.

As we flew on my pleasure grew and my eyes were glazed with delight and wonder when the biplane whispered onto the grass at Lebert.

There could be no stopping me now. I lived and slept flying, and within a year I had my pilot's license, and I earned two years of college credits in night aviation classes.

I was transferred to the Scott AFB Link Trainer section where I was appointed an Air Force Instrument Flight Simulator Instructor at the age of seventeen.

It was a time when things were going so well for me that I thought the next logical step in my life should be marriage. Family has always been important to me, and I married a girl of sixteen from the hills of Kentucky.

We both were too young and too inexperienced with life to know what we were doing, but Lillian Paradine Fuqua was a wonderful, unspoiled product of the hills and during our brief union, we were blessed with a son, Steve, who made the short marriage worthwhile.

Not long afterward Lillian and I moved on to new lives, and when I left the Air Force, I found myself torn between two loves, flying and broadcasting.

There weren't any great jobs in aviation open, and I soon found myself on-the-air in the small town of Dawson, Georgia.

Breaking into the broadcast business wasn't easy, but I had determination and luck. After failing an audition at WALB-TV and Radio in Albany, Georgia, the manager promised me a job if I could get six months on-air experience.

Of course it was the age-old question, which came first the chicken or the egg? No one wanted to hire you without experience, but how were you going to get experience without someone giving you a job?

I convinced the management of WDWD in Dawson to let me hang around on the weekends, without pay, and learn the business. After a few weekends of cleaning up the studios, watching and learning, the manager let me start by announcing "station breaks."

He offered me a job if I would start as a salesman. I did, and soon I had my own on-the-air shift.

After six months of experience, I returned to WALB-TV and radio and took an astonished manager up on his word. Of course, he never thought he would see me again, and he had little choice but to hire me.

He did, but what a shift I worked! I came in at 5:00 PM on Friday as the booth announcer for the TV station until after the late news at 11:30 P.M. I returned five and a half hours later to sign the radio station on the air and stayed at the control board until midnight—a nineteen-hour shift without a break. My sister, Billie, who lived in Albany, brought me my lunch and dinner. I ate while I aired a network program.

I returned Sunday morning at 8:00 A.M., signed the station on the air, and stayed there without a break until midnight. This way my forty-hour-week was logged in three days.

It was tough, but it gave me the opportunity to get some experience and do some news writing.

I took correspondence journalism courses and three years later, I arrived at Cape Canaveral where a hot dateline was in its infancy.

Again my luck was with me. Within three months of starting as a local reporter, my experience in aviation helped me land the job of covering the infant space program for the NBC Radio and Television Networks.

TWO

"The Cape: The Early Days"

During the late 1950s and early 1960s Cape Canaveral was a sprawling gateway to the future. It was the most vital and the most intensely exciting place in the country. It was a flat sandspit that had been reshaped by the hand of man into a fascinating, unreal, and at times overwhelming pit of blinding lights and sense-stunning thunder.

It was also deceiving, for beneath the palmetto scrub and sand spread a finely woven network of cables and wires carrying impulses of energy, vital messages, and the electronic commands to initiate motions which, if they were successful, would give earth the ability to reach other planets.

But it was a time when young rocket engineers suffered more failure and heartache than they enjoyed success.

It was a time when I broadcast play-by-play reports of exploding, flaming giants crying out in sky-shaking waves of rolling thunder. It was a time I told radio listeners that these great rockets did not die only violent, screaming deaths. They did not die with a simple fall from the heavens; they descended under protest.

The ballistic missiles did not simply blow up. They did not yield their life energy without a struggle. No rocket ever just exploded in a clean firefall. The flame began in spurts, out from the arteries of fuel lines, from the great reservoir of tanks, in blazing globules and long fiery streamers. Jagged remnants of the missile's once sleek, clean form fell blazing toward an ocean which waited unfeeling, willing to accept the ones that failed to run the gauntlet of fiery thrust and the chain of gravity.

This was Cape Canaveral in the early days, a world of giant rockets, of fire and thunder, and of nights exploding violently into days as men huddled within the protection of thick steel and concrete blockhouses, peering through periscopes, each shouting lift off.

They were also days of successes. One day in 1956 famed rocket scientist Dr. Wernher Von Braun and his Alabama launch team rolled a Redstone rocket with an upper stage and satellite to the pad only to have it called back by a tattle-tale Air Force Colonel who went running to the White House.

President Dwight Eisenhower insisted that the use of a military rocket would detract from the peaceful scientific intent of an American space program. Instead, he ordered development of an entire new booster, the Vanguard, to loft a tiny 3.2 pound satellite in celebration of International Geophysical Year.

The Soviet Union had no such qualms. On October 4, 1957, millions around the world stood in twilight or early dawn, anxious for a glimpse of a slow pinpoint of light moving across the sky, its shiny surface reflecting the rays of the rising or setting sun.

It was called Sputnik, the first manmade satellite. Its radio emitted an eerie beep-beep-beep. People were both fascinated and frightened, knowing man had put it there and wondering where it possibly could lead.

Few eras of history have had such precise beginnings. You couldn't, for example, date the birthday of the Middle Ages, the Renaissance, or the Industrial Revolution. But at 7:30 P.M. Moscow time, on Friday, October 4, 1957, that tiny, tantalizing speck of light, that incomprehensible beep, marked the birth of the Space Age.

It began as a triumph for one nation, and a humiliation for another.

The first word came to Washington, D.C., late on an Indian summer afternoon, by way of The Associated Press news wire. Five bells, signalling an important bulletin, preceded the simple, dramatic report:

LONDON (AP) Moscow Radio said tonight that the Soviet Union had launched an Earth satellite.

The satellite, the story followed, was silver in color, weighed 184 pounds, was about the size of a basketball and was orbiting 560 miles above the globe at 17,400 miles an hour.

The impact of Sputnik was enormous.

Until then, the Soviet Union was considered a backward country of baggy-pants peasants. America was the world's unchallenged technological leader.

The satellite not only symbolized the emergence of the Soviets as a technologically advanced society, but, more important and more ominous, it demonstrated that Moscow had the means to deliver nuclear weapons across continents and oceans to the United States.

Dr. Von Braun was disgusted. His team could have launched an American satellite a year earlier. He called the White House to get permission to put his satellite in orbit. Again, permission denied.

The decision was to stick with the Vanguard, and in the panic that followed Sputnik, Vanguard was rushed to the launch pad at the Cape. But before it could be launched, the Soviets again stunned the world by launching Sputnik 2 on November 3rd—less than a month after the first satellite. It weighed more than one ton and carried into orbit a dog named Laika.

Desperate, American launch crews worked every hour of each day to ready Vanguard. They cut too many corners, and when the designated December 6 launch date arrived, it was another day of bitter humiliation for the United States.

With the world watching, the slender rocket rose two feet off its launch platform, shuddered slightly, burst into flames and tumbled to the ground in fiery destruction. The tiny, grapefruit size satellite was flung free of the wreckage and lay on the ground, beeping, a forlorn symbol of massive American failure.

Newspapers around the world proclaimed: "Stayput-nik," "Ike's Sputnik is a Flopnik," "Oh, what a Flopnik."

It was a bleak day for America. To the men and women on the street, the failure generated feelings of lost confidence, wounded pride, confusion—and awe at the Soviet space achievements.

President Eisenhower decided after the Vanguard fiasco that something had to be done. He called Dr. Von Braun. "Can you launch your satellite in ninety days?"

"We'll launch it in sixty," a confident Von Braun replied.

Six weeks later, on January 31st, 1958, the Alabama missile team delivered. The Redstone rocket with the upper stage hurled Explorer 1 into orbit. America's first satellite weighed just thirty-one pounds, but it discovered grand mysteries about the earth and it catapulted the nation into the space age and a fierce competition with the Soviets.

We reporters overused the term "Space Race" in all our copy as we grew with the new high-tech industry, perhaps feeling more important than we really were in the new, high-pressure arena.

Celebrities came to the Cape from all over the world to watch the rockets "go or blow" as we said in those days, and we found ourselves rubbing elbows with Hollywood stars, famous test pilots, and influential politicians.

More satellites followed Explorer 1 into space and, buoyed by success, Congress and the administration made several things happen. The defense budget was increased significantly, and military rocket programs were given almost a blank check. Most forms of government-subsidized research began to grow. The nation's education system was overhauled, and federal dollars poured into schools to help produce an unmatched generation of scientists and engineers who became the heart of the American space reply to the Soviets.

The Pentagon formed the Advanced Research Projects Agency (ARPA) to guard against further U.S. technological slippage.

And the National Aeronautics and Space Administration was born.

America was on the move, but it needed someone to

manage the new space effort. But who would lead? The
Army, Navy, and Air Force all sought the assignment, as did
the Pentagon's ARPA and the Atomic Energy Commission.

But James Killian, the new White House science ad-
viser, focused on the National Advisory Committee for Aeronautics (NACA), and obscure group of part-time scientific
consultants who oversaw a few federal flight-technology laboratories.

NACA possessed some of the best engineering talent in
the country; was under civilian control, which Eisenhower
preferred; was too little known to have been caught up in the
partisan politics; and was a stranger to the red tape of government bureaucracy.

This sleepy little agency got the job of challenging the
Soviet space lead.

Reconstituted as the National Aeronautics and Space
Administration, the agency drew under its umbrella NACA's
five laboratories and 8,000 technicians; the California Institute of Technology's Jet Propulsion Laboratory; the Navy's
Vanguard project; and the Army's 4,000-man Von Braun
rocket team. Congress insisted the Pentagon maintain a separate space effort.

On October 1, 1958, a year after the Sputnik jolt, NASA
came into existence, but the "spook" boys around the Pentagon weren't happy. Much of the spotlight had been taken
away from the military, and even though the Air Force,
Army, and Navy were launching satellites, there was a question of size.

The Soviets had been hurling large satellites in orbit
and our efforts were puny in comparison.

The Advanced Research Projects Agency came up with a
propaganda scheme of launching a huge satellite, an Atlas
rocket itself, into orbit.

The Atlas was, at the time, the country's leading inter-
continental ballistic missile, and for it to hurl a warhead
more than 5,000 miles, the stage-and-a-half rocket had to almost achieve orbital speed. Engineers figured if they
stripped an Atlas, a so-called "hot rod" rocket, it would go
into orbit with the assist of the earth's 1,000 mile per hour
rotation.

The mission called for a launch due east, out of the range safety guidelines, but Major General Donald Yates, Commander of the Air Force Eastern Test Range, told the White House he could handle that.

Only eighty-eight people were brought in on the plan of placing a tape playback device and a small transmitter inside the Atlas' nose cone. The tape would play, over and over, President Eisenhower's voice wishing the world Seasons Greetings from space.

It was a grand publicity plan to one-up the Russians, and just in case it didn't work, the "spook" boys agreed the world would never know. They would never admit it had been tried.

The scheme was given the name "Project Score," and Atlas-10B was stripped for a flight on December 18th, 1958.

The mission was the most secret ever, and the "spooks" were off and running, but they made one little mistake. Two days before the launch, I was in a stall on a commode in the men's room down the hall from Major General Donald Yates' office when I heard a man with a familiar voice enter the room with a companion. It was the General himself, talking to an ARPA man.

"Check the place out," General Yates ordered.

The ARPA man looked around and took a peek under the stall doors. By then my feet were up around my waist and it appeared no one was using the facilities except themselves.

"My biggest concern is," Yates said to the ARPA man, "some damn reporter will get wind of this before the launch."

"So what?" the ARPA man questioned. "If he tells the world, and we fail, we'll simply deny it. He'll be left out on a long limb."

"Right," Yates said, "but if we get Ike's Christmas message in orbit, then the President can announce it himself from the White House."

"He'll be at some damn dinner," the ARPA man said.

"That'll be a good place to announce it," the General agreed.

The two men left the rest room and I sat there, wondering what the hell they were talking about.

The next launch was Atlas-10B, and I had read in an Air Force document how an Atlas almost achieved orbit each time it was launched.

That figures, I thought. They're gonna' orbit something with the Atlas. Something with a message from the President.

I forgot about the business at hand, and was quickly out of the stall and on my way to see a few solid sources, but because only eighty-eight people were in on the secret, everyone was in the dark.

Finally a high-ranking source within RCA, makers of the tape playback device, came through for me and I had the whole story. But as the "spook" said, there was little I could do with it except film the launch and standby for the announcement by the President.

I talked with Jim Kitchell, our Producer of Space News in New York, and after comparing notes, cameraman Bruce Powell flew in from Chicago.

Atlas-10B roared from a dark earth at 6:02 P.M. December 18th, 1958, and climbed into the rays of a sun that had already set below the horizon. For the first time I saw the most beautiful launch a person can witness.

In the virgin darkness, Atlas-10B's flame was deep red as it rose, faster and faster. But, suddenly, it was free of the early night. The line of shadow cast by the earth stretched far over our heads, but Atlas-10B was rushing from night back into daylight. Abruptly, the rocket and her fire trail were struck by a sun already well disappeared beyond the horizon. First the flame became a blood color, then a rich orange with increasing height, then an aurora grew to fill space, a multi-colored growing balloon in space as Atlas-10B disappeared over the horizon on a precise course to the east.

Its heading of ninety degrees was giving the big rocket all of earth's rotational push to get it into orbit, but it was also giving the "Range Safety Officer" in the control center fits.

The Air Force Captain kept trying to push the destruct

button as Atlas-10B flew farther and farther off his safety charts, but General Donald Yates stood over his shoulder with a firm grip on his hand. "Don't push the button, Captain," the General ordered. "I'll take full responsibility."

"But, Sir," the safety officer protested, "if we have a failure the missile will land on uncharted land in Africa."

"Big deal," the General bellowed. "So we'll kill a few damn tigers."

Atlas-10B flew safely on into orbit and the press reported it as a routine launch. I didn't report anything. I cut a sound track on the film and Bruce Powell was off to Jacksonville to process the film and standby for an 11:00 P.M. feed if the whole scheme was a success.

The Air Force returned the news media to Headquarters Building 425 at Patrick AFB where we had left our cars, and everyone was off to the bars, believing the story was over.

Major Ken Grine, the Information Chief, decided to stay in his office, and I decided to stay there with him. I had told him earlier what I knew, but he refused to comment. We both knew what we were waiting for, and a few minutes passed 8:00 P.M. it came. Directly from the White House. Confirmation by the President and suddenly the world was listening to Seasons Greetings from Ike transmitted from space.

NBC News was the only agency with film and we enjoyed our little exclusive, and, after five months on the job for the network, I ended the year satisfied.

It was the beginning of a high-pressure career that was not very intelligent for a person with my family history of heart disease, but I was only twenty-four—a time in a person's life when he or she believes death comes only to old people, never to the young.

I lived in a beach apartment with a studio, and life was good.

I had made many new friends, some of them even famous, but I suppose the one I liked most was a wild New Yorker named Martin Caidin. He was at the time, and still is, the greatest aviation and space writer around, and his books were very much in demand.

He lived in White Plains, and after he finished writing a book, Piper Aircraft would give him a plane and he would be off to the Cape for a little R & R (Rest and Relaxation). Just how a wise-ass New Yorker like Caidin could get along with a thick-headed Georgia plow boy like me was a mystery. But I reasoned it was because Caidin was an orphan and we both grew up with very little, grateful for what we had.

The night before I had been up late at the Cape covering some routine launch. Suddenly, only minutes after sunup, I was awakened by the roar of an aircraft buzzing my apartment and the shouts of a wild man in the air. I ran to my balcony to see this sleek Piper Tri-Pacer streaking over the beach, a head sticking out with a Texas bullhorn pressed to its lips. "Barbree," the shout echoed across the sand and waves, "come out with your hands up. We're not taking any prisoners. You're surrounded."

"Good Lord," I spoke quietly. "It's Caidin."

He waved the bullhorn at me and I waved back as I watched him fly away, westward toward the Merritt Island airport. I smiled. Good times were here.

I didn't know it then, but later I would write my first book with Martin Caidin: BICYCLES IN WAR. I would also help him research many of his books on space while we wrote EXOMAN, a made-for-television movie for Universal, and, also for Universal, I would write the SIX MILLION DOLLAR MAN episode PILOT ERROR.

Marty created Steve Austin, the SIX MILLION DOLLAR MAN, and wrote MAROONED, which became a major movie by Frank Capra starring Gregory Peck. What little I know about writing, I owe to him.

But these were the early days, when we were young and eager to party, and the next day Caidin and I were off to Miami Beach, flying the Tri-Pacer.

As a former instrument flight instructor, I didn't appreciate Caidin's takeoffs. He would climb the Tri-Pacer about 1200 feet per minute, just a couple of miles per hour over stall speed, and I was only comfortable with 500 feet per minute ascent, with a greater stall-speed margin.

"Get your nose down," I yelled at him during our climb to cruising altitude.

"What's wrong with the way I fly?" he bellowed in response.

"You'd make a damn good taxi cab driver, not a pilot," I yelled back, "Get your nose down."

"Okay," Caidin grinned. "From now on you make all the takeoffs."

"You got a deal," I said flatly. "A two-year-old could make a better takeoff than this."

It was a friendly argument, an understanding between two friends, and the Tri-Pacer hauled us safely down the coast to Ft. Lauderdale's Executive Airport.

After landing, we had trouble renting a car. There was only one left at the airport. A four-cylinder Rambler that was hitting on two. We could only get it to run about thirty miles per hour with the accelerator on the floor, but we took it anyway and made it to our hotel on Miami Beach.

Our friend Milt Sosin worked for the Miami News, and we thought it would be a good idea to give him a call so he could line us up with a couple of nice females to take to dinner that evening.

But there was a problem. We couldn't find Sosin, and Caidin had to spring into action. He came up with some of his books to impress the doorman. The smiling man told us to go upstairs, get dressed, and on our way out, he'd have a couple of dates ready for us. They were secretaries from Brooklyn and were guests in the hotel.

The two secretaries were also looking for evening companions, and, as promised, when we were ready to leave the hotel, they were there, waiting.

Soon Marty, I and our dates were off to do the town in our speedmobile, a Rambler hitting on two.

I was driving the rent-a-wreck north on Collins Avenue when a sleek, new Corvette pulled along side. A young man was at the wheel, minding his own business, when Caidin started his act.

"You think that piece of crap you're driving there will run, huh?" Caidin shouted.

The driver of the Corvette ignored him, and when the light changed to green, the sports car left us like we were growing in the cement. But, as luck would have it for Caidin, we caught the Corvette at the next light.

"That was nothing but luck," Caidin shouted to the driver. "My man wasn't ready. I know this Rambler looks and sounds like a piece of crap," he egged the sports car driver on, "but it will outrun that piece of Detroit trash any day."

Suddenly, the women with us were having second thoughts, but when the light changed, I slapped the accelerator to the floor, and the Rambler responded with a weak cough. The Corvette left us in our tracks and vanished over an elevated bridge. Caidin was laughing his head off in the back seat as I managed to get all two dangerous cylinders to push the Rambler to the top of the bridge and start our roll down the other side.

At the bottom, on the side of the road, sat the Corvette in front of a Police car.

Caidin's laughter could be heard across the nearby Everglades as we passed the officer writing the ticket.

"You're bad," I laughed over my shoulder. "You'll get yours, Caidin."

Minutes later we were in the Luau Restaurant on the 79th Street Causeway, drinking Polynesian cocktails from hollowed-out coconuts. The little umbrellas poked our noses and eyes each time we tried to take a drink. But, as we soon learned, the little umbrellas weren't our only problem. The drinks were very potent and, as people not used to drinking, Caidin and I were snockered within minutes. Even after the food arrived, the drinks kept coming and so did the jokes.

As our laughter grew in loudness, the maitre d's glances grew more stern. But we were beyond the point of caring. We reasoned the four of us were in a place we were not known so let the good times roll.

By then the jokes were coming so fast, and I was laughing so hard, that my eyes began to tear. I reached for my handkerchief and as I was wiping my eyes dry, Caidin looked suddenly stunned. With a sober face, and a sincere question, he asked, "What's wrong, Jace? Why are you crying?"

I realized he was serious and as I watched our dates' happy expressions change to concern, I seized the moment. "I really shouldn't be here having fun like this," I told them. "We buried my grandmother just last week."

"Oh, Jace, you didn't tell me that," Caidin moaned with more concern and the women nodded, adding their sympathy.

"She was ninety-eight, bless her," I said, the tears now rolling freely down my face.

"Ninety-eight?" Caidin questioned. "But, Jace, she had a very long life."

"Yes she did," I shook my head in agreement, "but thank God, they saved the *baby.*"

Caidin's face was a blank portrait frozen momentarily in time until he suddenly realized they had been had. He threw his arms straight up, his chair giving way, as he fell backwards onto the floor.

Suddenly every patron in the Luau was staring at this wild man, flat on his back, swinging his arms, kicking his legs, and howling with laughter.

The maitre d' walked over, looked down upon Caidin. "May I help you, sir?" he questioned sternly.

The hysterical Caidin stabbed a firm finger toward the maitre d' and repeated, "Thank God, they saved the baby."

Of course, we were invited to leave and we did, driving off into a night of memories best left untold.

We slept most of the next day, arriving at the airport at sunset where, in spite of our world record hangovers, we checked the Tri-Pacer, filed our flight plan, and soon Caidin had us rolling down the runway for the takeoff.

I was sitting in the right seat, and I quickly found the window seal a comfortable place for my throbbing head. I would have been grateful if someone would have shot me, but I had decided to tough it out when I suddenly felt the Tri-Pacer lift from the runway only to settle back on the concrete again.

Puzzled, I looked up to see the wind tee off to my right. I felt the plane lift again, bank to the right, and head straight for the wind direction device.

"Jesus Christ, Caidin," I shouted, turning to see Marty's head planted firmly on the left window's seal. "What kind of takeoff do you call this?"

He lifted up his head which was also suffering the agony of a hangover and said matter-of-factly, "I'm not making the takeoffs anymore," he grinned, "you are, remember?"

"God, what a madman," I laughed, reaching for the yoke, bringing the aircraft under control.

I flew the Tri-Pacer to our assigned altitude and took a northward course toward the Cape. The sunset over the Everglades was pink and gold and we tried to enjoy it in spite of our hangovers.

By the time we reached the Cape Canaveral area, the night air was calm and the Tripacer rock-steady. A pair of binoculars performed wonderfully in the clear air, and suddenly Cape Canaveral was spread out through the glasses, marvelously distinct and unbelievably close. Where the brilliant searchlights converged, an enormous missile stood. It was too far away to make out details, but I could see the plume of escaping liquid-oxygen vapor flashing in the light. The bird was sharp and clear, the launch complex brighter than day.

The Cape was a fairyland of lights and colors. Red, green, white, blue, cobalt, orange, yellow, all manner of lights, glowing steadily, blinking, flashing, moving. It was a riotous kaleidoscope, a Disney World of illuminated technology. We could make out along the northwest beach the four massive towers for Atlas, and the dark shapes where engineers and construction workers were rushing the completion of four complexes and their towers for the mighty Titan. There were the three towers for Thor, and that Intermediate Range Ballistic Missile's special family of Thor Able and the Lunar Probes, known as Thor Able I, II, and III. Through the glasses it was easy to identify the Jupiter, Redstone, and Jupiter-C complexes, and the new launch pad for Polaris.

I smiled to myself. Before the week was finished, I would be covering the first Polaris launch, the first solid-fueled missile designed to go to sea aboard nuclear submarines.

There were other areas too dark to identify from the air, but I realized I was seeing the Cape as I had never seen it before, and I further realized I was not merely seeing a site where buttons were pushed and missiles screamed into the sky. I was seeing a vast assembly, the workshop of a laboratory that stretched more than five thousand miles across the Atlantic. It was vibrant, expensive, terribly complicated, dangerous, but vital to all of us.

I turned westward, cutting power and trimming the Tri-Pacer for a rapid descent. Three brilliant lights flashed and disappeared, first white, then green. They were the flasher beacons from the grass airstrip on Merritt Island. I made a long, straight-in approach to the field and the Tri-Pacer settled easily on the grass. The flight from our lost weekend was over.

Our hangovers passed, and Marty Caidin returned to New York, and for Polaris' maiden launch, it was a beautiful Florida day.

The news media were brought onto the military range to better our working conditions. We were taken to the roof of a building a couple of miles from the missile's pad with the understanding that our phones would not be opened until ignition.

All went well with the agreement until shortly after liftoff. The stubby Polaris was the first solid-fueled missile launched, and the safety people had placed a destruct package on board that was used for liquid-fueled rockets.

The problem? The explosives used to destroy a wayward liquid-fueled missile were not destructive enough to destroy a solid-fueled rocket, and shortly after it began to fly, Polaris decided to go its own way.

The "Range Safety Officer" in Range Control sent a radio signal to destroy the missile. Instead of blowing it into harmless fiery debris, the destruct device only separated the Polaris' two stages, and the Cape squawk box carried an overly-excited voice screaming, "All personnel on the Cape take cover."

We stared into the sky above us, and we watched as the second stage of the Polaris tumbled our direction; the first stage, still burning, heading inland, across the adjoining Banana River and possibly Merritt Island.

I reached for my phone. The line was dead.

"The phones, Ken, turn on the phones," I yelled to our escort officer, Major Ken Grine.

"Get off this roof," Grine yelled back. "There'll be no phones."

"That's breaking the agreement," I protested, refusing to move.

At that very moment, a naval commander was bringing a tray of sandwiches for the press up the stairs, unaware of what was happening. A panicked Major Grine didn't give a damm about the phone agreement, or the sandwiches.

"Damm'it, follow me," he screamed, racing down the stairs, literally running over the naval commander.

With tray and sandwiches tumbling to the ground, Grine's only concern was for the press' safety. He was trying to get an organized group of fools to take cover.

We didn't move. Cameramen wrapped their legs around tripods and photographed the Polaris stage. Suddenly the big solid rocket plunged to earth a couple of hundred feet away with fiery debris falling all around us. One chunk hit the roof of a car and plunged through the Detroit steel to the floorboard.

The sight struck our consciousness. We had to record it. We were simply not concerned for our own safety. The story came first, and we watched the Polaris' first stage head inland, toward what appeared to us to be the city of Rockledge.

Hundreds could soon be killed. Again we demanded phones. None were open. We demanded to get off the Cape, to regain our freedom, and we were loaded onto the bus.

Next, when we went through the gate, I leaped from the military vehicle to the safety of civilian soil and ran for the first public phone. I was on the air within a minute, telling what I knew, and when I had completed my report, I ran into the highway, physically blocking the first car coming my way.

The driver gave me a ride to the Hitching Post Trailer Court, where crowds gathered. In the Banana River behind the rows of trailers, a cloud of steam burst from the water. The Polaris' first stage had slammed into the river. No damage was done.

I stopped long enough to catch my breath, to give thanks no one had been hurt, before I began interviewing members of the crowd.

But the talk among the eyewitnesses was not about the wayward missile, it was about the lady in a nearby trailer who had been taking a shower when the Polaris landed. She ran out to see what was going on and had forgotten one important item. Her clothes.

The Polaris was not only the first sea-going missile, it was also the newest member of the war rockets called IRBMs (Intermediate Range Ballistic Missile). IRBM meant the missile could hurl a nuclear warhead 1,500 miles.

My buddy Al Webb, the reporter at the Cape for the United Press International wire service, and I got together the following evening, and with our handy carpenter tools, fashioned a crude sign that read:

WATCH OUT FOR STRAY POLARIS
IBRM
"In the Banana River Missile"

Folks, I'm here to tell you the Pentagon has no sense of humor. Them folks can be as mean and nasty as U. S. Marshalls, and our sign wasn't appreciated. Its life lasted less than one fun-filled hour.

In that era the Cape was not only a young and exciting place; it was the site of a modern day Gold Rush. It was

Columbus' voyage to the New World, and it would soon be where astronauts would step into space; where for the first time man would head for another body in the solar system: Earth's natural satellite—the Moon.

THREE

"Astronauts and Other Assignments"

The young space agency knew from the beginning that its efforts must include a manned space program. The Soviets were heading in that direction, and on April 6th, 1959, I was heading for Wright Patterson Air Force Base in Dayton, Ohio.

NASA had decided its astronauts would come from the ranks of military test pilots. Fifty-eight Air Force, forty-seven Navy, and five pilots from the Marine Corps applied, and they were all undergoing extreme physiological, psychological, and leadership tests at Wright Pat.

My good buddy Jim Kitchell who produced space coverage and directed the Huntley-Brinkley report, asked me to join him at Wright Patterson. He was there with a Chet Huntley Reporting crew. He had been given permission to undergo the same tests as did the astronaut candidates.

Soon we were all there, and I was holding a microphone, trying to say something that made sense while I was being frozen, roasted, shaken, and isolated in chambers so quiet my heart's beats sounded like a High School base drum.

I did twelve reports for the "Monitor" network radio show, and we were there when the seven Mercury Astronauts were selected in Washington on April 9th, 1959.

Their names became legendary. From the Marines, Colonel John Glenn, and from the Navy: Lieutenant Com-

manders Alan B. Shepard, Jr., Walter M. Schirra, Jr., and
Lieutenant Malcom Scott Carpenter. From the Air Force:
Major Donald K. "Deke" Slayton, and Captains Virgil I.
"Gus" Grissom and the best and most "gutsy" pilot in the
world, L. Gordon "Gordo" Cooper, Jr.

The first thing Jim Kitchell and I decided to do was see
if any of the seven lived at Wright Patterson. We were in
luck. Captain Virgil I. "Gus" Grissom did, and Jim sent me,
the crew, and Producer Bill Hill out to the Grissom home.

Time was short. We needed an interview with an astronaut's wife for the evening's Huntley-Brinkley Report, and
when we reached the Grissom home, we leaped into action.

I stuck a microphone in Betty Grissom's face and asked
her, "How do you feel about your husband going into space?"

She didn't answer. She just sat there and looked at me.
"What do you want me to say?" she finally asked.

I smiled. "Just tell us how you feel about your husband
riding a rocket into space?"

Betty returned my smile and explained: "The two boys,
Scott and Mark, and I have been living with a test pilot. I
don't really feel flying into space is going to be all that different. She went on to say she felt it would be risky, but if that's
what Gus wanted to do, then she was all for it.

Well, she was right about one thing, that's what Gus
wanted to do, and when he got his first flight, riding the
Mercury capsule Liberty Bell Seven on a sub-orbital hop, he
made one request of engineer Sam Beddingfield. "Give me a
parachute."

"Good God! Gus," Sam exclaimed. "A parachute won't
do you any good. If the capsule's main chute doesn't open,
you won't have time to get out the hatch and pull the rip
cord."

"Oh yeah?" Gus laughed. "It'll give me something to do
on the way down."

Well, we got a good piece of film that day with Betty
Grissom, but before we could leave, we had to go out back
and shoot film of Mark Grissom's fox hole. He wouldn't have
it any other way, and we barely made it to our affiliate station in Dayton in time to get the film processed so that we
could get a report on Huntley-Brinkley.

The crew had problems getting the film processed and cut, and our report was quick and ragged.

In my part of the country, when a boy reaches his teens he is introduced to the adult world with a "Snipe Hunt." That's where he is taken into the woods at night, given a large sack to hold, while everyone else spreads out in the thicket to drive the "Snipes" his way, into the sack.

Of course, he's left alone, holding the bag, calling, as instructed, "Here Snipes, here lil' Snipes."

The others, laughing, spend the rest of the night wagering on how long it will take the "teen" to wise up, to come home with his sack under his arm.

Well, I soon realized I had just been taken on a New York City "Snipe Hunt," and I was left *holding the bag*. Every ragged element of the report was blamed on me, and I quickly learned that in television there was, and still is, a code: PYOA (Protect Your Own Ass).

The Mercury Seven moved to Langley Research Center in Virginia where they began their intense training while Vice President Lyndon B. Johnson, head of the space council for President Kennedy, got busy getting his oil buddies in Texas to donate some pasture land to Rice University.

They did, and Rice offered the land to NASA for a Manned Spacecraft Center, provided the space agency would construct all the buildings so they could be used as a university campus when the center was closed.

On the surface, it seemed like a fair deal for all, and no one talked about the fact NASA had 88,000 acres of land on Merritt Island, Florida where it built its launch center—a launch center that could only be located when a tracking range and other launch facilities were in place—a center with necessary equipment that just happened to be duplicated by the Mission Control Center.

To this day, the Houston center, now named after Johnson himself, is one of the biggest political "flim flams" that's ever been forced on the American taxpayer. But it was the "Space Race" and in those days all NASA had to do was go up

to Capitol Hill with buckets to haul back all the money they
wanted.

Even President John Kennedy committed the nation to
go to the moon before the 60s decade was out, and the Mercury Seven Astronauts, instant heroes to an admiring public,
were committed to climbing on board a rocket that may or
may not have been able to fly.

The Mercury capsule was about the size of a phone
booth and famed test pilot Chuck Yeager, who broke the
"sound barrier," laughed at the seven and called them "Spam
in a Can."

But the Mercury Seven were committed to make it
work, and they lived life on the edge, enjoying wild times in
wild cars. In fact, there have been so many stories told about
the original seven, it's difficult to separate facts from legends.

As a person who lived part of that history with them,
I'm here to tell you the nation's honor was well invested in
the group. Most of us admired them, and most reporters
watched out for their welfare as sports writers did for the
great Babe Ruth in the 1920s and '30s. The Mercury Astronauts would not survive in the circus-like atmosphere created by today's news media.

Even then, some sleaze newspapers and magazines
were constantly trying to get some dirt on the group, and the
seven's legendary infidelity didn't help their own cause.

One afternoon a sleaze-bag private investigator came to
my office with a tape. It was a recording of one of the astronauts in bed with a local gal who was well known on the
Cocoa Beach strip. The P.I. had bugged the room and the
"pillow talk" was very damaging to the Astronaut. It was for
sale and I suggested he leave the tape with me so I could play
it for my New York desk. The dumb P.I. left me his only
copy. I promptly erased it.

If the astronaut had been involved in stealing from the
taxpayer, endangering his mission, or putting anyone at risk,
then I would have led the pack in making his actions known
to the public. But, at the time, the country had a President
that made infidelity a national sport, and I wasn't about to
make an astronaut pay for a judgement in morals that did
not affect his job, or his committment to the country.

When I returned the tape to the private investigator, and when he later discovered it was blank, I played dumb. "Some stray radar signal must have erased it when you passed an antenna along the highway," I said, and the stupid P.I. bought it.

I never told the astronaut involved about the incident, but somehow I think he knew by some of the things I heard he later said about me. Anyway, I like to think he did.

On May 5th, 1961 Al Shepard made America's first space flight, a fifteen-minute sub-orbital hop that was duplicated July 21st of that year by Gus Grissom.

But unlike Shepard's picture-perfect flight, Gus had to swim for his life when his capsule's hatch blew prematurely in Bahamian waters.

"I was lying on my back, minding my own business," he told investigators later. "Pow! The next thing I knew, I could see blue sky, and water was coming over the sill."

Grissom struggled through the opening and into the Atlantic. His space suit was waterproof, but in his haste to get out, Gus forgot to close an oxygen hose port at his waist.

"Water was coming into the suit and I was getting lower and lower. It was hard to stay afloat," he told reporters later.

What he didn't tell reporters was that he had loaded his suit's legs with several pounds of dimes for souvenirs of his flight. The coins came close to drowning him.

Well, Gus didn't drown, and after their flights he and Al Shepard were the most well-known astronauts. They both loved to race the identical Corvettes General Motors provided for each of the Mercury Seven.

One night Grissom out-ran a local cop and wheeled the 'vette into the parking place before Al Shepard's motel room. Shepard had left his Corvette parked a few doors down, and Grissom slipped into his room.

The cop reached the motel a couple of minutes behind Gus. He simply checked for the 'vette with the hot hood, and promptly knocked on Shepard's door with the speeding ticket.

In another such legendary tale, the two astronauts speeded through Daytona Beach in Gus' Corvette.

The story goes that Gus told the cop who pulled them over that he was Astronaut Gus Grissom. It is said the cop replied, "Oh, yeah, I'm Alan Shepard."

"Oh, no you're not," Shepard said, leaning forward with his famous grin, "I am."

On another day the Astronauts' Corvettes were again involved in mischief.

Mercury program director Walt Williams was a serious man. Everything about Mercury was pioneering, the latest in high-tech theory, and the quiet man moved about the Cape shrouded in seriousness.

Williams was at the launch pad and he needed to be at a meeting off the Cape but he didn't have a car. Alan Shepard told him, "Take my 'vette, Walt, I'll catch a ride with Gus or John."

"That's great," Walt said, rushing from the pad, and driving away in Shepard's gray Corvette.

As soon as Williams made his turn onto the main road, Shepard phoned Cape security, and shouted, "This is Astronaut Shepard, someone just stole my Corvette. He's headed for the south gate."

When Williams reached the gate, security guards physically lifted him out of the car. They wouldn't listen to a word he said.

Walt Williams wouldn't speak to Shepard for weeks.

Less than a year after Alan Shepard made his historic flight, John Glenn became as popular as Shepard by making America's first flight into orbit.

John, who today is one of the country's leading United States Senators, was known as the "old boy scout" among the group, the clean-cut Marine who wouldn't do anything to tarnish his or the Astronauts' image.

John Glenn, in my opinion, is truly one of the finest people I know, but he is human.

Legendary launch pad leader Guenter Wendt likes to tell the story about how they got John going one time. "All our tests were pretty long and the first Mercury spacecraft didn't have a window. It only had a periscope.

"So I liven things up a bit by holding a picture of Playboy's centerfold for the month in front of the periscope. The doctors in the blockhouse went crazy because they couldn't figure out why John's heart and respiration rate went up so suddenly."

Henri Landwirth, known in the early days as "the innkeeper of the astronauts," survived one of Hitler's concentration camps and came to this country to become one of America's finest citizens. Today, he is in partnership with Senator John Glenn in some motels and he heads the "Give The Kids The World" group which makes sure many children with terminal illnesses receive their most fervent wish.

The night before Gordon Cooper's record-breaking 22-orbit Mercury flight in May 1963, the second group of astronauts—Tom Stafford, Pete Conrad, Frank Borman, the guys who would fly most of the Apollo moon landing missions—were joining the program and they came to Landwirth and asked him if they could throw a little informal dinner to meet the Mercury Seven.

They did. They prepared a dinner of breaded veal, deep fried, and potatoes. The veal turned out to be breaded cardboard and the potatoes weren't cooked.

Landwirth laughs and says, "Can you imagine sixteen astronauts sitting around a table trying to cut into cardboard?"

Of course, Gordon Cooper got a mouthful of the fried, paper cutlet but if indigestion bothered him he didn't tell. The next day, he was off on the most precise, the longest, and the most rewarding of the Mercury flights.

In the movie "The Right Stuff," the director kept trying to make Dennis Quaid, who played Cooper, say that the best pilot he had ever seen was the man who broke the sound barrier, Chuck Yeager. The truth is, L. Gordon Cooper, Jr. was the best of his day.

There are many stories about *the* Astronauts, some of which never happened, but a wise man once said, "When fact disputes a hero's legend, print the legend."

Well, I can't accept that, but I am in sympathy with the thought because I'm reminded of how quickly heroes are forgotten.

When the Grand Floridian Hotel was opened at Disney World in 1988, some of the Astronauts were there—Gordon Cooper, Al Shepard, Deke Slayton and John Glenn.

We were at an outside barbecue and Al Shepard was in the line for food which was located beneath the loud band.

The Master of Ceremonies stopped the music, and said, "Ladies and Gentlemen, we are very fortunate to have with us tonight one of America's outstanding heroes."

We reporters, astronauts, and most at the surrounding tables were sure he was going to point out Al Shepard, America's first man-in-space, the fifth person to walk on the Moon, a man who headed NASA's astronaut office for many years.

The M.C. continued. "Recording artist Clyde Fuddpucker, ladies and gentlemen."

We were stunned. This idiot not only had Al Shepard passing near his feet, he had hundreds of people in his audience that were far better known, had done far more for their country than some rock & roll recording artist.

Al returned to his table and as he passed I offered to get him Fuddpucker's autograph.

I suppose our time was like every generation's time. You had to be there with those seven young men. You had to be part of it, to know the guts it took to ride a rocket built by the lowest bidder, to spit in death's eye. To this day, when you speak about *THE* Astronauts, old timers in the space family think only of the Mercury Seven. All others are simply astronauts with little *a*'s.

During these exciting days I was married on September 3rd, 1960 to Jo Ann Reisinger, a person obviously too good for me.

All our friends agreed I married much better than Jo did, but nevertheless our union held firm.

The New York desk sent me chasing other stories in the southeast, including covering labor leader Jimmy Hoffa. In fact I first met the infamous labor boss in Federal Court in Orlando following the day we brought our first born, Alicia, home from the hospital.

As young parents we made a large mistake. We thought baby Alicia was so beautiful sleeping the day away that we never considered what would happen when we wanted to go to bed.

Alicia decided it was day instead of night and I went off to cover Jimmy Hoffa's court appearance with toothpicks propping my eyelids open.

Hoffa was in court accused of misusing pension funds, and it was just the beginning of his many legal problems. He had told a young, rich attorney by the name of Bobby Kennedy to go to hell. What Hoffa didn't know at the time was Kennedy's brother would be elected President and Bobby would be appointed Attorney General.

By October 1961 the push was on. Hoffa had been indicted not only on pension fund violations but also on jury tampering charges.

The following year when his trial on jury tampering was underway in Chattanooga, I was about the only reporter to whom he would talk. When court was over each day, Jimmy had a chest full of steam and a head full of gripes. He would come to where my crew had set up the camera, and we would let him have his say, blow his stack, and he would then answer NBC's questions. Film was cheap, and, of course, we used what we thought was news.

Some television types used what has become to be known as the "Sam Donaldson" approach. Hoffa knocked one of them on his ass outside of the Chattanooga federal building, and if that wasn't enough to endear him to most, he knocked a federal marshall on his ass too. The confrontations brought applause from those watching, and the labor leader simply made his way to our waiting NBC crew.

The truth was, Jimmy Hoffa had reason to be angry. He was being "railroaded" inside the courtroom.

Oh, I'm not saying Hoffa was innocent, he sure as hell wasn't but FBI agents would signal U. S. Attorneys when they didn't want to answer a question, and the government's legal hounds would bark an objection. The judge would rule in their favor, and the press would snicker.

The trial reminded many of us of the story going around in those times about blacks trying to register to vote in Alabama. As each applied, he was handed a newspaper and told if he wanted to vote, he must be able to read.

Stunned blacks would simply give up when they saw the paper was a Chinese publication.

But one voter registrar picked the wrong man. "What does that paper say?" the voter registrar asked.

The man met his eyes. "It says there ain't gonna' be many black folks voting in Alabama this year."

Jimmy Hoffa's jury tampering trial was much the same. There was no way he was going to get a fair trial, and even when he offered evidence that Bobby Kennedy was out to get him, no reporters would listen, and the judge wouldn't permit it to be entered into evidence.

In those days, the press wasn't going to print anything that put the Kennedy's, in a bad light.

For example, I was on an assignment backstopping our White House Correspondent in Miami when reporters were suddenly attracted to a commotion at the bottom of the lobby stairs of a hotel where President Kennedy was staying. A pretty blonde stood there crying.

White House staff people were trying to move her along, out of the public's eye, but she would not budge. "I want you people to know," she cried, "the President didn't like me. He wants a brunette," she said with disgust, resisting the tug of a large man.

"What's wrong with me?" she protested, throwing her breasts forward. "I've got as much as any damm brunette—a hell'va lot more than Jackie!"

The secret service boys moved in and physically removed her from the lobby. No editor touched the story, but today evidence of the young President's infidelity has appeared in many publications and on many TV reports.

Also, today, no editor would permit his politics to influence his news judgement, and certainly no one would sit still while any President appointed his brother Attorney General.

But Jimmy Hoffa went to jail, deservedly so say most, and now one of the biggest stories around is waiting for the reporter who uncovers what happened to him.

I'm not saying I approved of Hoffa's tactics. He grew up hungry and mean, and fought his way up the ranks of the Teamsters. But the man did have a sort of tough honesty. I got the feeling if you played it square with Jimmy Hoffa, you could expect the same treatment in return.

He once looked at me and said, "Barbree, you seem like a fair bastard." Then with his tight smile he quickly asked a question, "Does your mother know what you do for a living?"

Of course, we all laughed, but I had the feeling Hoffa was serious. Until you have been run over by a stampeding herd of reporters, you don't know what it is like to be thrown out in the street and stripped naked of every private thought and personal thing you may have ever possessed.

The news media as a whole is made up of a membership of nice, dedicated people. But we tend to run in packs, and if you are the prey, God help you.

FOUR

"The King That Was A Giant"

Sprawled in my seat, my long legs extended as far as they could reach. My head rested on the seat back, and I was worn to distraction from the bus pounding pavement. I was just tired of traveling, tired of my nose fighting the smell of drugstore lotions, unwashed skin, diesel fumes, tired of sucking into my lungs the same air breathed by thirty-odd passengers. Just tired of moving down a highway hour after hour.

I was on the bus because on May 4th, 1961, the day before Alan Shepard took America's first hop into space, thirteen blacks and whites left Washington, D. C. to take an integrated bus ride through the South. They were on a mission to integrate interstate buses, including the restrooms and restaurants in the bus stations.

The thirteen rode through Virginia, North Carolina, and Georgia without trouble, but when they reached Anniston, Alabama, the bus was bombed and burned.

The so-called Freedom Riders took another bus for Birmingham, and when they arrived, they were attacked and beaten by a mob. Two weeks later, another bus ride was organized for a trip to Montgomery.

A few reporters were invited to come along and the New York desk thought I should take the NBC seat. I boarded the bus and there I was with a load of excited young blacks and young northern whites who seem to think they were on a Sunday afternoon outing.

They were carrying signs that they would hang out the bus' windows through each town—signs that read:

"The Law of the Land is our Demand"
"Freedom's Wheels Are Rolling"
"Enforce the Constitution"
"End Segregation Now"

We rode along trouble free, and I wasn't wishing for anything different. I just wanted to get to Montgomery, call the desk, and hear the words, "Go back to the Cape, Jay."

The closer we got to Montgomery the more noise the kids made, singing protest songs and boasting they had won a victory.

I turned again to the window to watch a grove of pines flash by, tree trunks slashed deeply to drip white sugary sap into tin cups. A few miles later we passed a collection of ramshackle cabins with rusty tin roofs, floating wispy smoke tendrils from sagging chimneys. A turpentine camp. I'd seen plenty of them growing up in Georgia.

The roar of the bus flushed a big hawk and I watched the dark bird speed away along a narrow creek. I had a glimpse of brown waters spreading behind buildings on the outskirts of the capitol city of Alabama. Almost there, I thought, as the bus driver began to slow our speed, beginning his drive through city streets.

The demonstrators, both black and white, were singing louder now. They too were glad the ride was nearing its end. They were mostly college students, and, possibly for the first time in their young lives, they were feeling they had accomplished something important.

As the bus approached the station I peered forward and saw men crowding the streets and pavement around the building. The sun bounced from the windshields of pickup trucks spread in a manner to block traffic. Two or three dozen men stood loosely on the pavement, dressed in a mixture of overalls and denims. One man, standing in the front, wore straight khaki and held a whip. Suddenly I had a clear view of the whip man's real size. He was enormous, his gut overlapping a wide leather belt with a heavy silver buckle.

The driver turned to his passengers. "I don't know what this is," he said, the words coming nervously. "But I think we'd best unload here, and you kids best make a run for the station."

"I'm not afraid of these crackers," a white demonstrator boasted, leaving his seat for the door.

The others followed, singing, "Freedom, freedom," as they left the bus.

I picked up my tape recorder and followed the demonstrators through the door in time to see the whip move in a blur, to hear leather crack, to watch it slice a shirt, expose the shoulder of the white kid who challenged those he called *"crackers."*

Suddenly, the atmosphere was filled with screams and the protesters threw their signs down, ran toward the station with the mob after them.

I jumped from the bus, unthinking, and went for the fat man with the whip. He turned toward me just enough for my tape recorder to land squarely on his cheekbone. The blow snapped back his head and I stepped in close, driving my left fist into his stomach.

Suddenly, I wished to God I hadn't. The man staggered back, only one step. *That was all.* I might have just pushed him for all the damage I had done.

A huge arm plowed the handle of the whip into my face, knocking me against the front wheel of the bus. I felt the sharp edge of lug bolts grind into my back, tasted salty blood on suddenly loose teeth as my limp body sought the support of pavement.

My heroic efforts were finished as quickly as they had begun, and the fat man with the whip sought other prey. The attack by the mob continued for what seemed to be the longest minutes of my entire life before the police moved in and took some amount of control.

It was the third attack by mobs on civil rights protesters in Alabama within a month and Attorney General Robert Kennedy sent 400 U. S. Marshals to Montgomery to maintain order.

The following day, Dr. Martin Luther King, Jr. arrived in town and called for a mass meeting that evening in Montgomery's First Baptist Church.

The first of the big Civil Rights stories of the 1960s was underway in Montgomery, and I sat with the growing ranks of reporters who were occupying a couple of front pews.

I turned and studied the church. The walls outside peeling white paint, inside mildewed and grey with age; windows of stained glass, many chipped and broken; the choir loft filled with black faces and black bodies clad in robes of white. It was an old and large church, the kind that must have pleased God with all its smooth wearing of wood by kneeling knees.

I watched the crowd swell. All pews were now occupied and, at the rear of the building, more people were pushing in, standing, shuffling together.

Suddenly the murmuring noise that had filled the large church for an hour dropped away. It was a signal, a sign, and we watched as an elderly man stood behind the pulpit, his muscles establishing his frail but sinewy old body in a stance.

The instant we heard the first words of the old preacher, we were surprised by his strong voice and how his words could be heard. His message was part speech and part song . . .

". . . the Christ here to save us, to help us repent. We must cast out the Devil from our souls. Our Lord Jesus . . . cleanse yourselves . . . love your brother . . . peace for . . ."

The tempo of response by the crowd was quickening. My own pulse quickened with it. The older people rocked with the reading of the Scripture, mumbling aloud with it, not as the prophecy of some vanished era but as the stuff and staff of their living flesh.

". . . the humble shall be lifted up . . . the crooked shall be made straight . . . the mighty shall be brought low . . . in that mornin' Oh my Lord . . ."

From the choir loft the white-cassocked choristers sang out with a harmony that filtered through the dim light and bounced off the stained windows.

". . . for he knows, oh yes, he knows, just how much we can bear . . ."

"Sing it," the crowd breathed back and forth, male and female, here and there. "Sing it for Jesus!"

The old minister bowed his head in prayer once more, "Dr. Martin Luther King is the man, oh Lord, the man you have sent to lead us out of Egypt."

"Yes, yes! Yes, yes, it's so!" A moan sounded from one of the elderly women, swiftly hushed. Another moan broke loose. A heavy-set woman staggered to her feet. She fought against restraining hands to reach the aisle. Up front, another woman rose up, white-dressed, her hair knotted under a black hat. Her scream shattered the air.

I felt the hair on my head stand up. My very scalp lifted, tingling, and the choir broke into song, into Dr. King's favorite:

> *"When my way grows drear, precious Lord, linger*
>   *near;*
> *"When my life is almost gone;*
> *"Hear my cry, hear my call, hold my hand lest I fall;*
> *"Take my hand, precious Lord, lead me home."*

The choir finished and suddenly there was abrupt silence. The Reverend Dr. Martin Luther King, Jr. and his entourage walked heavily, purposefully, down the aisle, their heels thudding into the floor. It was the only sound in the church. Not a voice could be heard. The appearance of *the* man commanded the moment. They strode to the front of the church, to where their feet became tangled in wires and cables, the harsh lights illuminating them from the side.

Dr. King brushed the television cables aside and moved behind the pulpit, gripping it with both hands, and he looked straight ahead, across the large crowd of about a 1,000 people.

"Brothers and sisters, now is the time to be calm," Dr.

King's words were measured, strong, and they bounced off the altar, the stained glass windows and beyond, and echoed from the walls to reach every person in the church. "Now is the time to rise up without violence, stand firm for what is right, help your white brothers and sisters understand we are all God's children."

He thrust out his hands in stiffened posture, on his toes, hurling words of non-violence at them, feeling the words being picked up, held aloft, swept adoringly from hand to hand, crushed and hugged and kissed, and they sent the words back on a wave of thundering voices that rocked the building.

I was stunned. I had never heard anything like it, and I knew I was seeing something beyond the ordinary pale of human events. I was stunned because I discovered my own mouth open, felt my own feet stamping the floor and had caught myself only an instant before shouting with the rest. Good Lord! That man was alive with fire!

"There is something ugly outside this house of God tonight," Dr. King told them. "Something ugly and mean, but we are not going to join in the ugliness."

What the man in the pulpit was referring to was a mob of white segregationists gathering outside the church. They too were singing and yelling and growing in number while a squad of U. S. Marshalls and Montgomery policemen stood between them and the 1,000 blacks inside.

"We want to integrate, too," a strong voice rose above the mob.

"I wanta' go to church."

"Yeah, me too," another man yelled. "We all wanta' go to church."

I had moved outside as did most members of the press and we watched as the mood of the white mob grew more angry, tested the ranks of the police and marshals.

A bullhorn was lifted to the lips of a police captain. "You

people are ordered to disperse, to leave the area," the nervous symbol of authority said.

"We're not going anywhere," a man shouted, his voice rising above the noise of the mob. "Except, maybe to church," he added with an ugly laugh.

The man's defiance moved the mob behind him, and feet shuffled forward, ominous in their silence through which could be heard the clanking of bricks and bottles, and the soft slap of wood in hands. Then, with the ranks solid, not a word was spoken. The two forces stood before each other, poised on the brink, and that instant I found myself thrust into the emotional maw of the mob, and I was instantly aware of the absence of personalities. Faces vanished, names forgotten; all individual identity fled. Each group had seized upon the flesh of its numbers to emerge in startling birth as a sentient creature unto itself. Two hulking behemoths head to head, eye to eye, authority on one side, a way of life on the other, unblinking, on the edge of the abyss.

The man in front of the mob held a hand aloft and the arm swept forward as he uttered an unintelligible scream, releasing the tide behind him.

The white mob surged forward toward the church, the momentum of the front ranks impossible to check because of the shoving mass behind. The line of police and marshals waited, and then a barrage of bricks and bottles was rained on the church, and the police captain shouted through his bullhorn, "Gas 'em."

The white mob fled from the stinging clouds of tear gas, split into smaller mobs, and began taking its anger out on anyone nearby.

The press was an instant target. Axe handles went up and came down in chopping blows. Chains went back and around and whistled through the air toward their victims. The closed fists thudded home, heavy boots smacked sickeningly into unresisting flesh. Skin tore loose from bodies and splattered with crimson spray. Bones snapped audibly. Teeth were spat away from blood-choked throats. Fist and club and chain and clawing fingers.

The film rolled smoothly through the camera gate. Laurens Pearce grunted with self-satisfaction as he listened to the whine of the big Auricon. God, but he'd *never* shot film like this! It was a dream, impossible, but there it was, framed through the eyescope. Panicked reporters stumbled and lurched in pain and fear, trampling through hedges, staggering about cars on the street. A hell of a shot there; ah, that one. He zoomed in for a closeup of a pickaxe handle chopping down in a blurred arc. What a hell of a shot! The camera caught the wood cracking a skull, splitting flesh.

Glass shattered. Where the hell's the light, damnit! The lights, you stupid—Pearce turned, his outcry dying in his throat as he saw the pickaxe handle smashing the bright floods from the hands of his electrician.

"Git that television camera!" A hot cry of rage and even before he turned Pearce knew he was the prey.

Tag, and you're it, buster.

A solid wall from the mob bore down upon him, and Pearce hurled dedication to the winds and started running for his life. But he'd been in this game a long time and you just don't leave your camera. You try, damnit, you *try* to save your equipment. The camera was heavy and he threw all his strength into movement. He was still building up speed when he knew that he couldn't make it and—something jerked him forward. Nutto! God bless you, Paul, for the way his soundman was pulling on the umbilical cables connecting the camera to the sound amplifier. But he knew it might not be enough for safety. Not with that maddened herd of human buffalo pounding down upon them. He had a glimpse of even Nutto giving up the ghost, throwing away his sound equipment and sprinting madly toward the rental station wagon.

Throw away the camera, an inner voice shouted. It's too heavy, you fool. What the hell's the use of a camera if you're dead? But he couldn't. He staggered on, chest burning as he sucked in air, legs weak and rubbery, throwing all his strength into his desperate flight. The station wagon . . . just ahead. There; Paul Nutto opening the door. "Hold it!" Pearce gasped. "Hold it. I—" He stared in horror as Nutto staring at him with wide, fearful eyes slammed the door shut, cowering on the seat. This was the moment when he thought of Nutto as a wide-eyed bug to be squashed and—

Oh, God, the pain. A chain walloped into the camera, several links curling around to slice open his ear. He felt the harness jerk, his knees giving way completely and his body pitching helplessly toward the ground. Protect yourself. He twisted and looked up. Just in time to see the second chain looming huge as it slammed lengthwise into his face. Liquid fire erupted along his cheek and lips and nose and his eyes and what was white became spraying crimson. "Jesus Christ, that's my blood!" he cried out to no one, to everyone, astonished he was cursing instead of screaming, and his fingers clawed at the harness buckle to free himself from the imprisoning weight and bulk of the camera. He rolled clear of the chain. There! Got away from—A heavy boot banged into his ribs and he knew something had broken. He felt his eyes water and was dimly grateful that his own panic was stronger than the pain as he scrambled madly for the safety of the station wagon. *No! It couldn't be! Locked . . .*

He begged, pleaded, beseeched. "The door! Open the door, for God's sake!" he screamed at the fear-paralyzed Nutto, hunched on the seat like an animal. No answer. But redemption was there. A hand jerked him away from the station wagon as if he was an empty sack of clothes. A heavy boot dropkicked him in the groin and through the savaging of his body and soul he felt the warmth trickling between his thighs. If only he could scream. If only he could die. But there was no breath, only pain, and—his mind froze, locked solid, as a thumb started into his eye socket, and he knew he was helpless to prevent that thumb from splitting out his eyeball like a bloody grape and—

"That fella's had it." A voice from somewhere. The thumb slid away. Someone delivered a final kick for fun to his groin. It missed and thudded into his lower stomach and

with a feeling of utter dismay worse than the pain he knew
he was soiling himself.

Pearce lay more dead than alive on the ground as the
door opened slowly. He stared through one eye as Nutto
knelt beside the bloodied cameraman, reached out with a
shaking hand.

Pearce retched, slipped in his own bile, felt the anger
still there, rushing adrenaline through his system. He raised
to one elbow, shook a pitifully weak fist at the other man.
"Paul, you son of a bitch," he gurgled through his own blood.
"If I live through this, I'm gonna' kill you."

"Damnit, Laurens," Nutto quivered. "Weren't no sense
in both of us getting our asses kicked."

The battle raged for most of the night, but inside the church
the blacks linked arms and sang, "We Shall Overcome."

> "Oh, deep in my heart,
> "I do believe . . .
> "We shall overcome someday."

The Governor sent in the national guard, martial law
was declared, and the mob was sent fleeing into the night.

During the coming months, demonstrators continued to
ride buses through the South, and the Interstate Commerce
Commission restated its original ruling that segregation on
buses and in bus stations was unlawful.

On December 12th, 1961, twelve so-called freedom riders were arrested in Albany, Georgia, the city where I
worked before moving to the Cape, and I was on my way
again to another Civil Rights assignment.

Dr. King and his staff moved into the city and planned
what would be a campaign against Albany's social and economic structure.

In Montgomery, Dr. King and his followers had been
arrested for disobedience of laws they felt unjust, and whites
had been playing into their hands. The whites would react

with anger, often beating the demonstrators, and the police would look the other way.

But in Albany, the chief of police saw to it that all demonstrators were handled with great care as they were taken off to jail.

One of Dr. King's tactics was to march down the street without a parade permit, breaking a local law, and Albany officials made sure they were on television cameras, begging Dr. King to accept a parade permit.

"We'll be very happy to grant you a parade permit, Dr. King," Deputy Police Chief Leslie Summerford said, offering the permit to the civil rights leader. "Just sign here, sir, and no laws will be violated. You are more than welcome to march."

But Dr. King refused to sign it. His tactic was to break the law, go to jail, hopefully with police roughing up the demonstrators. But this time it wasn't working. The police smiled, begged the marchers to accept the parade permit, and when they refused, they appeared to be the bad guys, not the police.

Dr. King sat in his jail cell with the Reverend Ralph Abernathy, his friend and the second in command of the Southern Christian Leadership Conference.

I had spoken to Dr. King before, interviewed him, but did not know him well. Dr. Abernathy was another question. He and I had hit it off, and had enjoyed several conversations when the word came that he and Dr. King wanted to see me.

Other reporters complained. I was being taken inside the jail for an exclusive interview, but Dr. King and Dr. Abernathy made it plain they wanted to talk with me off the record.

I agreed and was taken to their jail cell where two confused civil rights leaders sat, wondering.

"What's going on here, Jay?" Dr. King asked. "What are these people up to?"

"Yeah," Dr. Abernathy joined in. "You used to work here, right?"

"Right, I did," I answered. "They're basically good people."

"Good people?" Dr. Abernathy raised his voice. "How can they be good people? They're segregationists?"

"Segregationists, yes," I agreed, raising a hand. "But they don't practice segregation because of hate, they practice it because of tradition."

"Aw, com'on, Jay," Dr. Abernathy said, disgust in his voice. "They hate our guts."

"Oh, no they don't," I protested, rising slightly out of my chair. "They are closer friendships and trust between some blacks and whites here than they are between whites."

"How's that, Jay?" Dr. King asked.

"Dr. King," I turned directly toward him. "You don't eat the food prepared by people you hate! You don't trust the raising of your children with people you hate!"

"That's right," the man spoke gently. "But you're talking about servant roles here, Jay. You're not talking about engineers, doctors, other professional people."

I suddenly felt ashamed. "I understand, sir," I told him. "But it's not a black and white issue, if you will forgive the pun," I grinned, "but there's rights and wrongs on both side of the question."

"Well," Dr. Abernathy spoke up, "if these people are as good as you say, why are they fighting us?"

"Tradition!" I said. "It's that simple. *Tradition.*"

"Tradition, huh?" Dr. King smiled. "I still can't eat their tradition in one of their white restaurants."

I nodded, I understood. "That's wrong, sir," I said, "and most of these people here privately agree it's wrong." I shifted in my seat. "In fact, Dr. King," I continued, "many admire you, admire what you are doing, it's just . . ."

"Just what, Jay?" Dr. Abernathy interrupted.

"It's just that no one likes to be told what their mother and father taught them is evil," I stared at them. "That's what you are doing, that's what you are telling these people," I argued. "You're telling them their mother and father, their ancestors, all of their family were and are evil people. That just won't wash here or anywhere, gentlemen."

"Seems I heard this argument before," Dr. King said. "It seems I heard it from Indian friends, from Muslims, even from some of my Jewish friends," he smiled. "So, I know where you're coming from, Jay," he added, standing up, turning away from me. "When this struggle is over," he continued, "we are going to need men and women of good will from both sides, not just black and white, but from all cultures."

He turned back to me. "The world is getting too small, Jay. We must all learn to live together."

"That's the kind of thinking, sir, that has won you the admiration of most," I said firmly, looking directly into Dr. King's eyes and feeling his greatness. "But, I doubt if you asked me here to get my views on race relations," I added with a smile.

"You're right, Jay," he laughed. "Ralph here thought you might be able to shed some light on why our efforts here are failing."

"It's simple, sir," I said flatly. "You're not dealing with mean people. These folks simply are not going to mistreat you."

"It's as simple as that?" he questioned.

"Yes, sir!"

"I understand," he said, offering me his hand, "Thank you for coming."

I gripped his hand firmly. "My honor, sir," I said, turning to say my goodbyes to Dr. Abernathy as well.

As I left the Albany jail, I suddenly realized I had just had the honor of speaking to the man many blacks consider their Savior. It was that simple. Dr. Martin Luther King, Jr. was their Prophet, their Deliverer, and until we whites recognized that, there was going to be trouble between the races.

In Albany, Dr. King found no brutality and the federal government could not and did not intervene. He left the city defeated, but when the 1964 Civil Rights Bill was passed, Albany was among the first to integrate not only its public facilities, but its private restaurants and hotels and motels— a fact we noted on the Huntley-Brinkley Report.

Mean people in other cities did not disappoint Dr. King. He took his movement to Birmingham, back to Montgomery, to Selma, even northern cities like Chicago and Newark. He was even awarded the Nobel Prize for Peace, but the most violent city of his campaign proved to be the nation's oldest city, St. Augustine, Florida.

The year was 1964, and St. Augustine proudly displayed for all its tourists what blacks felt was a symbol of shame, an affront to them and their ancestors.

In a downtown park, tourists walked through a restored "Slave Market," and conditions for blacks in St. Augustine were as bad as they were anywhere in the land. It was a sort of segregation that hurt. That was wide open in its intent. The word "nigger" was widely used, and there were people who would instantly go on camera to explain how and why the white man was superior to the black man.

Most of my colleagues from the North referred to these people in their copy and on the air as members of the Ku Klux Klan. But they weren't the Klan. In fact there was no Klan in the city of St. Augustine. I told my colleagues this, but many considered me a bigot simply because I was from Georgia, and went about their work with closed minds.

I tended to my business, did my reports as accurately as I could, and finally one day during the St. Augustine campaign, I was asked by a reporter why I was certain these people weren't Klansmen?

"Simple," I answered. "They are Catholic. St. Augustine's population is mostly Catholic."

"So," he said. "They could still be Klan."

"Nope," I smiled. "Only WASPs can belong to the Klan. Only Protestants. No Catholics. No Jews."

"I'll be damned," he said, shaking his head. "I hadn't thought about that."

"Most people don't," I smiled again. "They just assume, they prejudge, and that's prejudice—the prejudging of something."

"Wait a minute," he held up a hand, protesting. "Are you saying I'm prejudiced?"

"Yep," I laughed. "You're prejudiced against prejudiced people."

The protest written on his face turned to a smile.

"Damn, if you're not right, Barbree," he said, his smile turning to laughter.

I laughed with him, not at him, and said, "Everyone prejudges someone or some culture. Westerners prejudge the motive of Easterners, and Arabs mistrust the Jews, and . . . you get the picture."

"Yes, I get the picture," he continued his laugh, "And I can see you are prejudging me now. You are prejudging my ability to comprehend."

"Well," I grinned. "You do work for the New York Times don't you?"

"Guilty," he said, still laughing.

The Times reporter brought his laughter under control and said, "This reminds me of something Will Rogers was suppose to have said."

"What's that?"

" 'What makes man ignorant is not what he doesn't know, it's what he knows that ain't so.' "

I had been in St. Augustine for three weeks when the "showdown" arrived. A youthful Andrew Young, the same Andrew Young who afterward was Ambassador to the United Nations for President Jimmy Carter's administration and later Mayor of Atlanta, was leading marchers from a black church to the "Old Slave Market" in a downtown park.

During the marches there had been scuffles between whites and blacks, but nothing compared to what had taken place in other Civil Rights campaigns.

Andrew Young was Executive Vice President of the Southern Christian Leadership Conference—a "right arm" for Dr. Martin Luther King, Jr.

Dr. King had been invited to St. Augustine, but Andy Young and other staff members had been sent in to get the campaign underway. And for three weeks, they had been skirmishing with local segregationists who were growing in number, and confident their actions would not be frowned upon by local law enforcement.

The storm had been gathering and *the* night was upon

us as Andrew Young led two columns out of the church, a
soon-to-be bobbling sea of motion, surging and ebbing in the
bright television lights.

I walked quickly along the side of the marchers, occasionally running to the front, then falling to the rear to make
sure I didn't miss anything.

Our crew kept in step as we listened to the voices, ragged but swelling, through the dirt street community. *"Ain't
gonna' let nobody turn me around, turn me around, turn me
around,"* a turntable of repetition, a sound of resolution, of
commitment.

They marched down the street, down the dirt sidewalks,
in front of a bar whose customers deserted the juke box,
crowded into the doorway to gape at Andrew Young and his
followers.

"Freedom,   freedom . . . ,"   their   voices   growing
stronger in the night air . . .

They shuffled their out-of-cadence feet by the pool room
where the familiar snap of cueballs ceased, where the arguments inside stopped abruptly while some stared, and some
ran outside to join the marchers' ranks.

"Before I'll be a slave,
"I'll be buried in my grave,
"And go home, to my Lord,
"And be free . . ."

Andy Young led them by the red-hot smell of sizzling
ribs in the Bar-B-Q and on past teeming shotgun houses
where blacks stood in astonished awe.

"Oh, deep in my heart,
"I do believe,
"We shall overcome,
"Someday . . ."

We watched the marchers turn right at the main street
to the downtown park and head for the "Old Slave Market."
We knew tonight would not be the same. Too many people
had been alerted, and each television crew began loading
fresh film for their entrance into the "whites only" world.

"Ain't gonna' let nobody,
"Turn me around,

"Turn me around,
"Turn me around . . ."

They marched into the park in a small tidal wave, self-contained, carrying in the audacity of its own forward motion the seeds of its destruction; for whites had gathered in the park, another group at the "Old Slave Market," and still another across from the park at the foot of the bridge. Others just sat in their cars and stared.

Andrew Young and his band were hurling the gauntlet, spitting in segregationists' eyes . . .

"Before I'll be a slave,
"I'll be buried in my grave,
"And go home to my Lord,
"And be free . . ."

They moved into the "Old Slave Market," in a tighter band now, ranks close together, feet shuffling, pounding together beneath linked arms and hands.

"I ain't gonna' let nobody,
"Oh, Lord,
"Turn me around, turn me around,
"Oh, Lord,
"Turn me around, turn me around,
"Oh, Lord,
"We're gonna' keep on a walking,
"Keep on a talking,
"Keep on a marching to freedom land . . ."

Andrew Young held up a hand, marking time, standing fast while his feet tramped up and down in heavy slow rhythm. Up and down, a dull thudding boom of hundreds of feet; pound, pound, pound. Behind the stopped front ranks the others shoved and pushed, wondering at the end of motion, eager to see what was happening. Young brought his hand down and with a crash of silence the thudding boom of feet ended. The youthful black leader surveyed the whites before him, his head turning slowly.

Suddenly, Andrew Young went to his knees in prayer. On the spot where blacks were sold into slavery one hundred years before, he began to pray as white faces moved toward him, cursing. Other whites stood gaping, disbelieving what they saw—a man in prayer being beaten.

There was no fight.

There was no struggle. In the midst of their torture, at the worst of the whites' cruel punishment, even as they were being punched and kicked, the blacks never forgot their quest. Their cry of battle was nonviolence, and they were sworn to their new religion, and as true soldiers the dark-skinned people followed their creed.

The front ranks staggered, buckled, collapsed, and fell in pain and agony. At once those immediately behind threw themselves forward, hurled their own bodies on Andrew Young and the other wounded to absorb the second and third and following blows.

The second wave of bodies collapsed willingly on the first to form a blanket of protection. They were beaten as fiercely, and the third wave rushed forward, arms and faces and groins and breasts and bodies open to absorb the blows. They protected those already hurt and more rushed forward like moths to the flame to protect the others. And still more, until the human mound was so large, the angry whites gave up in frustration and took out after reporters, and photographers, and television crews, and any blacks outside of the "Old Slave Market."

People, black and white, starting fleeing in all directions and I was no exception.

"There's one," a rough voice bellowed. "There's one of them Yankee reporters. Git 'im."

I stopped, turned, and took careful aim at the wall of screaming whites thundering toward me. "I'm no damn Yankee," I yelled, shattering my tape recorder into snuff-blackened teeth. "I'm from Georgia."

The man grabbed his mouth, wiped blood, and I had just one question. *Why in the hell did I do that?*

I thought about running again, but there wasn't time. With a savage cry a huge body leaped through the air, knocked me to the ground, burying my face in an immense stomach. The fat man smelled like something shot in the woods, a heavy, musky scent of hide and hair.

I felt other hands poking, punching and digging at me, and I felt myself smothering beneath heavy flesh. Suddenly the fat man was jerked upward, and I looked into a black sky. I was free. Between me and the mob was a flash of fists and flying hair. It was other whites—some of whom I'd seen operating downtown business establishments. They fought silently and with incredible fury until the mob simply opened up and vanished.

I leaped to my feet to say thanks, but as quickly as they had appeared they vanished, running to the aid of others.

I started to run again as I heard a vehicle's brakes squeal. I spun about. Bill Cavanaugh, our cameraman, in his rental car.

I jumped into the car as Bill did a tight, U-turn in the middle of the street. I slapped him on the back, "Let's head for the church, Willie."

Morning came with sore ribs, a few bruises, and the loss of skin and hair above my left ear. But I had fared better than most, and I set out to do something I should have done days before.

David Hunter was Press Secretary to Florida Governor Farris Bryant, and we were friends. We had even been in business together, operating a radio news service for a while when I was first stringing for NBC.

I phoned David and explained what was going on in St. Augustine; by nightfall there were two hundred fifty state troopers in town. Law was restored to the country's oldest city.

Years later, during the Jimmy Carter presidential campaign, I was on assignment with Governor Carter in the Watts District of Los Angeles, and we stopped long enough for refreshments at a local fruit stand. I found myself standing next to Andrew Young, and after I reminded him of that night in St. Augustine, he smiled and said, "I didn't feel a thing. It's surprising," he continued, "but I've looked at film after film of that beating, and I don't see how I wasn't killed. But," he shook his head, "I didn't feel a thing."

Of course, the violence during the 1960s didn't end in St. Augustine, it spread into the North, and I was sent to such places as New York City itself and Providence, Rhode Island.

I would later learn the reason I was needed in New York City where we had hundreds of reporters, was because most of them, even black reporters, refused to cover civil rights protests; and to keep the desk from calling them, they wouldn't answer their home phones.

What most reporters did was to install an unlisted phone and give the number to their friends and family. They simply ignored the rings of their listed phone during riots.

What really kept me sane during those days was being able to return to my refuge of Cocoa Beach, back to covering space, and spending quality time with my family.

Daughter Karla was born November 8th, 1966, when Dr. Martin Luther King, Jr. was turning his efforts away from the Civil Rights battles and leading protests against the Vietnam War.

Because of this, many people who had supported him, turned away and the news media lost interest. Even when he returned to marching for black causes, his day seemed to have passed. In April 1968, in the midst of a garbage collectors' strike in Memphis, Tennessee, he marched but few reported it or noticed.

But one rifle bullet would change that.

FIVE

"The Bullet That Almost Killed A Nation"

The air stinks. I took the corner slowly, my muscles taut. I glanced about to be certain the car doors were locked, every window jammed tight into its recess. My fingers curled tightly about the wheel. *The air stinks,* I said to myself again, and I was dismayed with the thought. My headlights swept along the building on the far corner, gleaming wet over garbage piled high because of the two-month-old garbage strike —garbage that had spilled along the gutter and into the street. I felt the tires crunch and grind their way over the mess, but that wasn't what I smelled. The air conditioning took care of the garbage, the animal excrement dumped along the concrete. The debris of this block and the others behind and still before me was as natural as broken windows gaping at the world from shattered tenements. *The air stinks from fear. Mine, and, theirs.* And I knew I was right. You don't mistake that electric sensation, when your nostrils flare and the adrenaline rushes through your system. I knew I was scared because of the way I gripped the wheel, the way I kept my right foot on the gas pedal, my left foot resting ever so lightly on the brake, ready for *anything.*

What had brought me to this world of anxiety had actually begun decades before, but the chapter of the present began mid-afternoon when a tall man with a long nose paid for a room at Mrs. Bessie Brewer's rooming house. The man

signed in as John Willard and went upstairs to Room 5—a
room with a window facing the Lorraine Motel.

The tall man sat down, opened a beer, and began sipping and watching. Watching Room 306 at the Lorraine
where Dr. Martin Luther King, Jr. was staying while he was
in Memphis. He was there to help lead the fight of the city's
garbage collectors. They had been on strike since February
12th, and this was April 4th, 1968.

Dr. King said dignity was the real issue in Memphis.
Blacks had won many legal rights, but the garbage collectors
were striking for economic rights, and he and other black
leaders were staying at the Lorraine Motel, laying out plans,
and pulling the movement together.

A couple of minutes before 6:00 P.M. Dr. King left his
room and stepped onto the balcony. He wanted some fresh
air before dinner and another of the endless rallies he had
held during the past decade.

The tall man in Room 5 in Mrs. Bessie Brewer's rooming house now held a sniper's weapon. He stood in the bath-
tub and steadied the rifle on the windowsill. He was 205 feet
away.

From the parking lot below, the Civil Rights leader's
driver called. "You best take a coat to the rally, Dr. King. It's
gonna' be chilly tonight."

"Okay, I will," Dr. King called back, lifting his arms
from the balcony's railing, standing straight up to begin his
return to his room.

It was one minute past 6:00 P.M., and the tall man in the
rooming house took a deep breath, his right hand squeezed
the rifle, his finger slowly pulled the trigger.

The bullet left the weapon, traveled the two hundred
five feet in a microsecond, and ripped through Dr. King's jaw
and neck. The tall man watched his target being snapped
backwards in a twisting motion, watched Dr. King crumble
onto the balcony. It was obvious a second bullet would not
be needed.

Dr. King's staff, and other motel guests, rushed to his
aid and the news of the assassination flashed across the
country, then around the world.

I was in an Aikido class (a Japanese method of self-defense) in Cocoa Beach when my desk called. In less than two hours, I was on my way to Memphis where I seemed to be driving the only car down fear-filled streets, on my way to the Lorraine Motel.

The news was already filled with rioting, with buildings being burned to the ground in cities across the nation, and here I was alone, driving through Memphis' streets occupied by blacks.

The garbage wasn't frightening me. Not that, or the run-down buildings, or the fact that my headlights were the principal source of illumination lighting the rotting canyon of scarred walls. What frightened me were the shadows. They were everywhere, dark skin melting into dark night. They were moving about, turning slowly, watching the car rolling through their midst, and they were wondering what in the hell is this crazy white man doing off his turf and on *ours?* Especially on this night.

The headlights slid along a gutted wreck of a car, wheels gone, windows smashed, a hollow travesty being left overnight in this neighborhood. More garbage beyond. Shapes moving quickly before my headlights. I resisted the temptation to slam the accelerator to the floor and just get the hell out of there at eighty miles an hour.

Someone jumped in front of the car. Instinct brought my left foot slamming onto the brake, and the vehicle jerked wildly, tires screeching. I had only a glimpse of white teeth flashing in a dark face, and in the same instant I heard the hands against the doors, pressing again and again on the handles to open the car. I snapped my head to the right, saw a hulking figure. Just at that instant a black fist banged angrily against the glass. Hammering by my left ear. Another shadow there, brandishing a tire iron, starting to swing. My foot tramped the pedal and the car bounded ahead, tires screeching on the asphalt, and in a swift one-two-three explosion of events, I saw the figure dancing lightly away from the fender, heard the tire iron clang dully against the rear of the vehicle in a useless motion of hate. Number three came a moment later, a brick sailing out of darkness, missing the front windshield because of my sudden movement, but slamming with a heavy thud on the roof. *A brick that was meant for me when I was dragged out of this thing . . .*

Rubber burned as I floored the accelerator, and through the closed windows and hum of the air-conditioning system I heard the tires scream. A night scream in Memphis. A jungle cry that brought the natives running quickly to the curbs to see what was going on. Telegraph system and there was a gauntlet ahead. Headlights moving quickly across young faces, heaving more trash through the air.

I spun the wheel wildly to the left. Too late. A heavy garbage can bounced from a stairway onto the sidewalk, clattered onto the street directly in front of my car. I managed to avoid hitting it head-on, but it thudded into the right front headlight and the light winked out. I thought I heard the glass breaking, but I couldn't be sure because the car still rang with the impact of the heavy can, and it rocked from side to side as I swerved back to the center of the street. My heart pounded inside my chest.

A huge spray of garbage whipsawed along the hood and slid greasily across the windshield. Suddenly I thought of getting a ticket for speeding and I laughed hoarsely at the thought. God, I'd welcome a cop right now. I'd welcome a whole legion of them. But they weren't here, and I pressed harder on the pedal, and the big car lunged forward. More figures dashed into the street, daring me not to hit my brakes. "Well, damm you!" I shouted, still racing along, my right hand banging again and again on the horn, swerving from left to right. The black figures taunted me with their lives. The one headlight of my car stabbed into the night like a lopsided Cyclopean beam and I knew if that light went out I wouldn't slow my speed but would take my chances by rushing on.

Just a few more blocks, I thought, and I felt the perspiration drenching me, felt the musk-stink of my own fear filling the car. A cab shot out of a side street. I slammed my foot down on the brake. The tires burned again, scorching pavement, the rear end sliding wildly for a few terrible moments. Then the cab disappeared, and I was safe. Suddenly the car's damned engine stalled. I shoved the gearshift into "park," turned the starter-key. Out of the corner of my eye I saw shadows coming, a loose assembly, moving confidently, *flowing* out of the darkness toward the car. I twisted the key savagely, cursing the car to start. I heard and felt hands at the door handles and at the same moment the engine caught and screeched with sudden power.

Numb, sucking air deeply into my lungs, I stomped on the accelerator and raced away from the dark streets, spun the car's wheels as I climbed onto an entrance ramp to the expressway, slid into traffic, and headed to my motel. My assignment The Lorraine Motel, the scene of Dr. King's assassination, would have to wait for daylight.

After checking in, I left my bags in the lobby, and slid into a booth in the motel's lounge, shaking slightly, the inevitable aftermath of what I'd gone through. The waitress brought me a double Jack Black on the rocks and stared with wide eyes as I gulped the sour mash whiskey. The heat spread through my system and I found myself getting a better grasp on my nerves. I handed the glass back to the waitress. "Make it another double," I said crisply. "I'll be right back." I went to a pay telephone, called the desk, told them I was in Memphis, and filled them in on my attempt to reach the Lorraine Motel.

"Get some sleep," Assignment Editor Al Buchard said. "All hell's broken loose tonight. They're burning Washington down."

"I thought we'd be in for it!"

"Just call in tomorrow, Jay," he said, hanging up before I could acknowledge his instructions.

Usually I can't sleep the first night in a strange motel room but the whiskey helped. I dropped off an hour or so later with the TV still carrying up-to-date reports on the aftermath following Dr. King's assassination. The night would prove to be the first of many before the country would learn to live with the loss of a large chunk of its conscience.

Morning came and I was only one of thousands of reporters who had moved into Memphis overnight. We took to the streets to learn what we could about the assassination that had touched off the most widespread rampage of rioting, burning, and looting this country had ever seen.

The trouble was not isolated to Memphis. Blacks took to the streets in Chicago, Baltimore, Detroit, and Washington, D. C. itself.

Federal troops moved into the nation's capitol city with fixed bayonets. Machine gun nests were put in place to protect the Capitol building, while troops surrounded the White House.

All across the country, blacks began to gather in the streets as they heard about the murder. They were devastated, angry, some moving about with hollow feelings locked inside, most suffering a loss almost too terrible to bear. But there were some who took advantage of the situation. They were not followers of Dr. Martin Luther King, Jr. Many were simply thieves, and many were called bums by other blacks.

These were the people who treated Dr. King's death like it was carnival time—time to frolic and have a good time. They smashed in store windows, grabbed television sets, anything they could carry, some stopping to try on a new jacket or a dress or a pair of shoes.

The trouble lasted until dawn, and after a few hours, as a new night approached, the looting and burning was worse. Entire neighborhoods were burned down, never to be rebuilt. No business person could afford the insurance.

Most blacks did not participate in the rioting and looting. They felt too badly about the loss of Dr. King, and they were good people, people that worked hard, made do on what they had.

We shot a piece of film of an elderly woman trying to stop a group of looters, begging them to stop. "Ain't we got enough trouble without you bums burning our neighborhood down?"

The weekend following Dr. King's assassination, seventy-two thousand Army and National Guard troops were called to duty across the nation, They had to deal with trouble in 168 cities. Twenty-four thousand people were arrested, forty-three were killed, but in spite of all the devastation, the country was spared a race war.

Law enforcement had learned much from handling riots during the four previous summers. Police, and military troops too, had learned that a single human life was far more valuable than any property.

Dr. King was laid to rest, and some tried to continue his movement. There was the "Poor People's Campaign," and beginning with my assignment to cover Dr. King's assassination and burial, I was away from home for three-and-a-half months.

After Dr. King, the Civil Rights Movement was never the same, and that fall I covered the Republican National Convention in Miami, and got ready for Project Apollo, the first journey of man to another body in our solar system—the Moon.

SIX

"The Moon and Beyond"

Late in 1968 the Soviets were busy readying a spacecraft to make a circumlunar flight with two Cosmonauts, a first-time feat that would have permitted them to lay claim to reaching the moon before the United States.

NASA officials looked upon their circumlunar flight as nothing more than a propaganda move to steal Project Apollo's upcoming thunder. Only men landing on the Moon, walking and riding on its surface, bringing back lunar rocks and other samples for geologists would be of any value.

NASA Officials were angry. They made the decision to send Apollo-8 to the Moon, to put it in orbit around the lunar surface during the upcoming holidays.

"Why Christmas?" I asked in a news conference. "Why not wait until the first of the year?"

"We're flying Christmas because we're ready," Tom Paine, NASA's acting Administrator answered me. "We're ready to take the next step forward in the nation's space program."

Of course, what I and other reporters did not know then was what NASA knew about the Russians' effort. The Apollo launch team was in a race with the Soviets and what began with Project Mercury, what took the lives of the Apollo-1 crew in the launch pad fire, was at stake.

NASA wasn't about to let what Astronauts Gus Grissom,

Ed White, and Roger Chaffee paid for with their lives be stolen by some cheap propaganda trick.

Everyone had come too far, given too much.

There was John Glenn's ride into orbit on a rocket built by the lowest bidder, followed by the flights of Scott Carpenter and Wally Schirra, and the final Mercury mission; the *pilot's* flight flown by L. Gordon Cooper, Jr.

Insiders knew that Gordo Cooper was the best pilot of the Mercury Seven Astronauts. He was called a "hot dog" by some, but called that with respect.

Insiders also knew Cooper had been held back because of the politics of the time. His Oklahoma twang did not project the image the Kennedy Administration wanted to create, and Cooper was held back, pushed aside for those without any ties to the South, with a region of the country that was under fire as responsible for most of the nation's social troubles.

NASA had decided to test the Mercury spacecraft to its limits and the agency set the project's final flight for twenty-two orbits—thirty-four hours.

On May 15th, 1963, during the final hours of the countdown, a calm and ready Gordon Cooper fell asleep sitting in his Faith-7 Mercury capsule on top of a fueled and volatile Atlas rocket. He had to be awakened for his ride into orbit where he would become the first Astronaut to sleep in space —a ride that went well until the 19th orbit.

Gordo had been in space a record twenty-nine hours when a green light appeared on the cockpit panel. The green light said the ship was heading back to earth. Like hell it is, Cooper smiled to himself as a concerned Mercury Control tried to figure out what caused it.

While engineers were trying to determine why the green light had appeared, trouble began to pile up. Electrical surges on orbit 20 knocked out the instruments that told Cooper the position of his spacecraft, and on orbit 21, power to Faith-7's automatic control system went out. If the Mercury capsule was to fly, Gordo would have to do it himself.

The most critical maneuver was firing the spacecraft's retro rockets. This had to be done with split-second timing, with the Mercury capsule in the most precise position. Just a micro-degree off, or a split-second early, or late, would mean Gordon Cooper's Faith-7 would splashdown hundreds of miles from its planned landing target.

The "hot dog," the best of the Seven, was being asked to perform as accurately as a computer, as skillfully as the best auto-pilot man could build. A lesser pilot would obviously fail. Gordon Cooper's chances were slim and none.

With just an hour to go in the mission, Mercury Control worked out the precise maneuvers required and John Glenn, the old boy scout himself, was stationed on a tracking ship south of Japan.

Glenn transmitted the numbers to Cooper and at that perfect, precise spot in space, Gordo fired the big retro-rocket pack. He was slammed against his seat, felt like he had stopped on a dime in space, but, instead, Faith-7 was on its way home. Right on track, precisely on the reentry flight path.

"It's been a real fine flight, Gordon," John Glenn radioed him. "Beautiful all the way."

Glenn was right, of course, but Cooper wasn't yet out of the woods. Ahead of him his flight skills would be tested again when the Mercury spacecraft slammed into earth's atmosphere at 17,000 miles per hour. A wall of fire and friction. A precise penetration needed to keep Faith-7 from burning up, from leaving L. Gordon Cooper, Jr. as black ashes floating gently to earth.

Cooper flew like he had never flown before. All of the skills his pilot father had taught him, all the books and great flyers could teach him in test pilot school, all the thousands of hours he had literally worn out high-speed aircraft in flight, had honed his abilities for this moment.

With just the right touch, L. Gordon Cooper, Jr. steered his Faith-7 through the searing heat of reentry and landed just four miles from his primary recovery ship, the U. S. S. Kearsarge. Computers before and since have not done better.

The master pilot would fly again. He would command the eight-day Gemini-5 mission with Astronaut Charles "Pete" Conrad in August 1965. But the best would not get a ride to the moon. A disagreement between Cooper and fellow Mercury Astronaut Donald "Deke" Slayton cost him any hope of walking on the lunar surface.

Slayton was in charge of the Astronaut Office. He was the one man who selected the crews.

Gordon Cooper retired.

Gemini was the bridge between Project Mercury and the Apollo flights. The project was designed to investigate in actual flight many of the critical situations that would be faced by the moon voyagers.

Ten Gemini missions were flown to develop procedures such as rendezvous in space, docking with other spacecraft, and how astronauts would adapt to the world of weightlessness long enough to reach the moon and return to the gravity of earth.

Four days before Christmas, 1968, the beaches and causeways in the Cape Canaveral area were jammed with tents, RVs, and parked cars. Nearly a million people gathered to witness history.

Projects Mercury and Gemini *were* history and all eyes were focused on Launch Pad 39A, where three astronauts had boarded Apollo-8 as the first human cargo for the gigantic Saturn 5 rocket.

This was no routine launch. This was an attempt to send three men a quarter-of-a-million miles from home on a risky mission to orbit a body in the solar system other than their home planet.

I sat at my microphone in the NBC News complex three and a half miles away, telling a world-wide audience what I saw before me. Not only was our broadcast carried on the NBC Radio Network, it was picked up by the BBC, British Isles, Armed Forces Radio, the Australian networks, sixteen broadcast groups in all.

What I saw was a thirty-six-story-tall rocket, the largest ever built, a giant standing alone with Astronauts Frank Borman, James Lovell, and William Anders sealed within its higher ramparts, umbilicals linking its flanks to the launch tower. A blizzard of ice and snow particles was falling onto the massive hold-down arms clamping the Saturn 5 to its launch stand.

At 7:51 A.M. on that clear Saturday there was a hush among the thousands at the press site when ignition began, a savage light tearing at our eyes. One moment, a giant waiting for life and in between one heartbeat and the next a cascade of fire leapt into being beneath the first stage. Few of us could follow the path of flame where it tore into thick, curving iron tubes deep within its launch pad, crashed into thousands of gallons of water and emerged from each side of the launch mesa as an orange-hued, swirling rupture of fire and steam over a thousand feet high.

Saturn 5 was alive.

A blizzard fell across the floor of the launch platform, a swirling glitter of ice shaken from its flanks. The seconds passed. Pressure built inside, flame raged faster, and then, a deep, groaning bellow; massive steel hold down arms snapped back and the Saturn 5 was free.

The giant, the mightiest of all rockets, rose slowly, majestically, its mighty power plant generating 7.5 million pounds of thrust. The thunder and the shock wave rolled back to earth, drowning out the applause and the "oohs" and "aahs" of the spectators.

All along the periphery of the blast zone, seventeen thousand feet from the launch pad, sound crashed against the onlookers with body-shaking impact. No mere thunder. No howling cry of the smaller rockets. This was too loud. The beat was too low a frequency. The shock waves of five colossal engines slammed together, an outpouring of sonic violence from diamond-shaped shock waves raced outward in all directions as a series of swiftly repeated bomb explosions, a crash of one blast after the other.

Inside our studio, objects not secured to the building's floor or walls shook loose, fell to the floor, rolled under tables and chairs and desks.

During the first launch of a Saturn 5, our next door neighbor's studio ceiling fell. Our neighbor is CBS. And the reporter under the crumbling ceiling? Walter Cronkite.

Moments later the huge rocket was over the Atlantic, the golden color deepened to orange and then violet-red along the edges of the flame. The giant no longer climbed vertically but programed in a long, curving assault upon the mass of the planet. The flame lengthened to a thousand feet, its trailing edges ethereal, expanding in a rush, lengthening as atmosphere thinned with every second. Then there was a huge plasma sheath, a glowing envelope of ionized gases out-pouring silently in the rays of the morning sun, and people for hundreds of miles up and down the Florida coast saw Apollo-8 head for the moon.

Eleven and a half minutes after the thunderous liftoff, the third stage of the Saturn 5 injected Apollo-8 into an orbit 115 miles above the earth—a vital first step in man's first journey for a close up look at the lunar landscape.

For nearly two trips around earth, almost three hours in time, the astronauts and mission control checked and rechecked every system, every piece of the hardware, making sure everything was perfect before committing themselves to fly away to the moon.

Flight controllers looked at each other. The flight director checked all their faces. There was a nod of agreement, a confirmation on the communications loop, and Apollo-8 Commander Frank Borman was given the go-ahead. High over the Pacific, the third stage was refired and it burned for five minutes. This continuous burst of power increased the spacecraft's speed from 17,400 to 24,200 miles an hour, and Apollo-8's crew became the first humans to break the grip of earth's gravity.

Borman, Lovell, and Anders were on their way, three days away from orbiting the lunar landscape, getting man's first look at the moon's darkside.

On their second day out, Commander Borman reported his crew had flu-like symptoms. Doctors on the ground prescribed sleeping pills and a diarrhea-control pill, and the next day all three felt better. What they didn't know at the time was in future flights, half of the astronauts in space would feel that way on their second day in weightlessness. Flight planners began planning major assignments on the first and third, and later days to give the crew time to get over "space motion sickness."

When Apollo-8 crossed the 200,000 miles from earth

mark, the astronauts sent back a television picture of their home planet. It was breathtaking. Part of the earth in shadow, part in sunlight, with great patches of clouds.

"For colors, the waters are all sort of royal blue," reported James Lovell. "Clouds, of course, are bright white. The land areas are generally brownish. What I keep imagining," he added, "is if I'm some lonely traveler from another planet, what I'd think of the earth at this altitude—whether I'd think it would be inhabited or not."

"You don't see anyone wave, do you?" laughed Mission Control.

Minutes after the astronauts signed off, Apollo-8 reached the "equigravisphere," the point where the gravitational pull of earth and the moon are equal. The spacecraft was traveling only 2,200 miles an hour. Its speed had diminished gradually, like a car traveling uphill. Now, less than 40,000 miles from the moon, Borman, Lovell, and Anders were now under the influence of another gravitational field rather than that of their home planet, and they were being pulled toward an orbit around the lunar surface.

Early on Christmas Eve, Apollo-8 sailed behind the moon's backside, and back there, Commander Borman fired the spacecraft's big engine, dropping Apollo-8 in lunar orbit. The firing was done out of radio contact with Mission Control, and when Apollo-8 emerged around the moon's edge, excited flight controllers on the ground knew the ship was in orbit.

Astronaut Lovell gave the first report on the moon's surface from seventy miles away. He described it as "essentially gray, no color. It looks like plaster of paris, a sort of grayish beach sand."

Lovell's report answered the first of many questions about that alien world which had awed man since the earth's beginning, and during the next twenty hours many more would be answered.

Apollo-8's crew took thousands of pictures of a wild and vacant landscape, and scouted landing sites for future Apollo astronauts before returning safely to earth.

The next flight to the Moon was Apollo-10, a final dress rehearsal for the big one, the first actual landing by Apollo-11.

A ghostly figure slowly descended the ladder. He hesitated carefully on the bottom rung, and then lowered himself onto the dish-shaped footpad of his landing craft.

One half billion people watched the history-making event on television on a planet a quarter-of-a-million miles away.

The ghostly figure carefully extended his left foot, reached beyond the lunar landing craft's footpad, and, like a swimmer testing the water, American astronaut Neil Armstrong planted the foot firmly in the lunar soil.

"That's one small step for man," he spoke, his words hesitant, "one giant leap for mankind."

Man first set foot on the moon at 10:56 P.M. eastern time, on Sunday, July 20th, 1969. It was a moment about which we broadcasters had little to say. The drama of that instant in time said it all, and I simply added, "They did it."

Astronaut Buzz Aldrin climbed down the ladder minutes later, and for about two hours these men of history explored the moon while enthralled earthlings watched.

I sat in our studio overlooking the Mission Control Center in Houston and said such things into my microphone as, "Centuries of dreams and prophecies have now come true. Man has broken his terrestrial bonds and set foot on another world. It is an exciting portent of the future. For beyond lie the planets and stars," and as I spoke the words, I had a certain knowing and understanding that one day my grandchildren would be participating, playing some small role in man's journeys to these distance worlds.

Apollo-11 was a major success. Armstrong and Aldrin's footprints on the moon would be joined by those of ten other astronauts, and Project Apollo would end as it began with a tremendous success.

It was a time when the country needed to see its flag on the moon, to see Americans there, to find in the astronauts heroes that were lacking in a country that had lost its pride and dignity in the jungles of South Vietnam—a country that lost its manhood in its streets filled with war protesters.

It was also a time when we paid little attention to diet, to our foul habits of saturating the air we breathed with tobacco smoke, and I surely didn't have the time to concern myself with such things.

Inside my chest, the cigarette smoke that was affecting my lungs' ability to function, and the fat-saturated blood that flowed through my arteries and veins, was slowly, but steadily, adding to heredity's construction of artery-blocking plaque within my coronaries. Of course, I didn't know it then.

It was a time we were certain we would live forever, and the success of Apollo bred celebrations, good times with drink and smoke and rich foods, and after each mission, those of us involved spent the night celebrating.

The "Splashdown Parties" were memorable but none would ever measure up to the excitement and destruction of Apollo-11's.

Chet Huntley, America's premier TV news anchor, was the most-loved broadcaster in those days as well as one of God's warmest and most considerate people. But, when Chet dranked, he changed from a nice introvert to an "everything goes" extrovert.

The night following Apollo-11's splashdown, Chet topped the evening off by pushing a piano player and, of course, her piano into the hotel swimming pool.

SEVEN

"Heart Trouble On the Moon"

Jim Irwin and Dave Scott fell toward the moon in a lunar module named Falcon, their eyes fixed on what they saw through the landing craft's windows.

They were quick to discover that looking down from space onto the lifeless surface, the moon held up a mocking face. The blackness of craters imparted false depth to the circular shapes; most lunar craters were in reality shallow, dish-shaped depressions, mere dents in a rugged and rippling surface.

Even where the great seas and plains seemed from afar level and smooth, change occurred with a steady pace. It was as if they were in a microscopic craft rushing toward the satiny skin of a beautiful woman; the closer they approached, the more glaring became the blemishes and faults concealed from the eye by distance. The apparently flat surfaces of the moon presented much the same changing view until it became obvious that before them floated the victim of a brutal game of celestial target practice, the results of billions of years of meteoroids plunging into its airless surface.

They fell steadily toward the moon, and the light playing on the lifeless landscape rippled with the shadowed interference of the Apennine Mountains, the fantastic canyon named Hadley Rille. This was the spot where they were going to land, but their landing site was hidden in the shadow of Mount Hadley, a lunar mountain twice as high as Colorado's Pike's Peak.

"Falcon, does it look like you are going to clear the mountains?" Mission Control asked.

"Houston, we've got our eyes closed; we're pulling our feet up," Dave Scott answers.

"Open your eyes. That's like going to the Grand Canyon and not looking."

They were down in a nine by forty-five mile orbit—that is nine miles above the average surface of the moon at their lowest point, but there are many lunar mountains higher than that.

They looked out on the horizon and saw high peaks; it felt like they were just skimming along. But they really knew they were moving fast, travelling at Mach 5—3,000 miles per hour.

"Falcon, stand by. On my mark, sixty seconds until landing sequence starts."

Jim Irwin tugged the cinches on his body harness, assuring taut restraint. His legs were spread slightly, booted feet evenly against the deck of the lunar module.

A quarter of a million miles away earth was the distant, lesser world, and Jim found that difficult to accept. The blue planet was a dazzling liquid globe suspended against velvet blackness. It commanded space, captured the center of the universe, and located in Mission Control were flight surgeons who had failed to diagnose coronary artery disease in the lunar module pilot's body.

None of the stress tests, none of their medical techniques had spotted the growing plaque in Jim's arteries that were little by little starving his heart of the precious blood it needed to continue pumping, beating seventy times a minute to keep Jim Irwin alive.

He was a quarter of a million miles and three days away from the nearest doctor, but in the excitement of the lunar landing, he hadn't the slightest hint he might need one.

"Falcon, Houston, thirty seconds."

The lunar module Falcon was just big enough for the two pilots to stand side by side and look out the window. The area to the rear was just long enough for a man to sleep.

Together they were landing on the moon with a living space smaller than a bedroom on a train.

Jim shifted within his space suit, applied elbow pressure to the arm braces at his sides, preparing for the explosive transition he knew was coming. It was almost time for the Power Descent Initiation Burn, twelve minutes of Falcon's descent engine burning to place them on the lunar surface.

"Falcon, Houston. Fifteen seconds."

Jim held his breath for the final moments before the descent rocket would be fired as Falcon slid along a flat angle toward its computed target. The interior of the lunar module glowed with soft electroluminescent lighting from the front and side instrument panels. Directly before him, in the center console, flight instruments and display gauges stood out sharply, a contrast of light against light. Through the triangular windows he could see the mountainous lunar horizon, sawtoothed against the blackness that lay beyond.

"Ten seconds, Falcon."

Jim glued his eyes to the glowing panels before him. Range and azimuth numbers glowed, changed, kept changing.

"Five seconds."

They were almost at the exact moment of firing. At that instant when the lunar module reached a point 192 miles from the landing target, when the lunar surface lay 50,174 feet below, flame would spear along his direction of flight. Blazing thrust to kill their forward velocity, keep them sliding moonward.

"Ignition."

The numbers flickered.

A tremendous blow struck the bottom of Jim Irwin and Dave Scott's feet. Flame lanced the lunar skies, sound clanged wildly through the lunar module. Braced as they were, still they sagged downward, dragged by deceleration grinding through their bodies.

They gasped, a mixture of severe pressure and excitement with the moment. They increased the weight on the grooved armrests, and their faces reflected a savage joy.

Jim reveled in the pressure clamped upon his body. His

muscles answered the punishment, compensated for the deceleration, and in spite of clogged coronary arteries, his heart hung in there. This was what he'd waited, struggled, trained, prayed for over a period of many years. This was prayers answered. The thunder of the descent engine was sweet music to his ears.

"Forty-two thousand, Falcon!"

The flame stabbed ahead of them. Deceleration built up as the lunar module blasted away its weight with the fuel gushing into the combustion chamber.

No sound carried down to the moon. Not a whisper of the blazing rocket engine reached beyond the cabin. Inside Falcon, thunder clanged and beat through the ship. Beyond the metal walls silence prevailed in airless space as it had done for billions of years.

"Twenty-five thousand, Falcon!"

"Roger, Houston."

The lunar pilots repeated the altitude and velocity changes to Mission Control as they flashed on the panel. Altitude changed slowly, distance swiftly in the arrowing descent. Speed fell off, a steady progression, a trade-off of kinetic energy for reduced velocity.

Lower, slower the lunar module moved, riding the mathematically precise rails of orbital mechanics.

Landing legs outspread for the feel of the moon's surface, the silver-and-gold machine knifed toward the mountain range that lay directly ahead.

"Twenty thousand, Falcon!"

The shadows stretched far across the lunar plains, lancing outward from the Apennine Mountains and high curving walls emblazoned with raw sunlight. Down they went, racing across the surface, descending more rapidly in a steepening arc, the pilots snapping out velocity, height, distance to their target, angle of descent.

"Ten thousand, Falcon!"

"Roger, Houston."

At 8,000 feet they pitched over, changing their altitude about thirty degrees. They had been coming in on their backs, looking up, feet first. Suddenly they had a good view of the landing site, and a good view of Mount Hadley Delta.

They were at 7,000 feet, and Mount Hadley was towering above them, soaring up 13,000 feet from its base. It gave them the impression they were a little short of their landing point.

They could see Hadley Rille, the great canyon, and they played the landing point to be about the right relative distance from it. There were lots of craters out there, and they looked for a smooth place to land.

Seconds later, Command Pilot Scott locked Falcon in on a landing spot and the lunar module was no longer moving forward. It was coming straight down.

"Dave, you've got a good spot," Jim told him, convinced they were going to have the smoothest, easiest touchdown of all the Apollo landings.

At about one hundred feet, the descent rocket and steering engines began to stir up dust. Suddenly they were consumed in the cloud of moon dust and were searching for the surface with instruments.

A probe on the landing gear would turn on a light in the cabin and tell them when to shutdown the descent rocket.

The probe light came on. Jim shouted, "Contact!"

Dave Scott shut off the rocket engine, and Falcon fell, hitting the surface hard.

"BAM!" Jim yelled.

The lunar module pitched up and rolled off to the side. It was a tremendous impact with a pitching and rolling motion. Everything rocked around, and they thought all the gear was going to fall off. They were sure something was broken and thought they might have to go into one of the abort situations.

If Falcon had passed forty-five degrees in its tilt, they would have had to lift off immediately. If the lunar module had turned over on its side, they would have been stuck on the moon.

The Falcon stopped moving, settled in its tracks, and Dave Scott told the ground, "Okay, Houston, the Falcon is on the plain at Hadley."

Flight Controllers in Mission Control quickly searched their consoles, read their instruments. The lunar module was okay. They could stay on the surface.

"Roger, roger, Falcon!" Mission Control acknowledged, the room filled with applause.

As soon as Jim and Dave received the STAY they began to power the Falcon down. They had landed on the rim of a small crater, but they were safe.

They pounded each other on the shoulder. Real relief and gratitude filled their smiles and feelings. They had made it.

Jim Irwin and Dave Scott looked across a beautiful little valley. The great Apennines were gold and brown in the early morning sunshine. Jim thought it was like some lovely valley in the mountains of Colorado, high above the timberline.

They would spend three days there, exploring a place where man had never been, and there were times when Jim Irwin looked up to see the earth. It was a difficult maneuver in his bulky space suit. He had to grab onto something and hold himself steady and then he would lean back as far as he could.

"That beautiful, warm living object looked so fragile, so delicate," he would later tell me, "I felt that if I had touched it with a finger it would have crumbled and fell apart."

Jim said that in spite of all the excitement of exploring the moon, seeing the earth from the lunar surface has to change a man, has to make a man appreciate the creation of God and the love of God.

Jim and his crewmates Dave Scott and Al Worden had brought a special plaque with them to the moon, a plaque honoring three Soviet cosmonauts who had died four weeks earlier. It was a reminder that space flight was anything but routine, that danger was always a companion.

The Soyuz 11 crew, Georgi Dobrovolsky, Vladislav Volkov, and Viktor Patsayev, gave no indication of trouble as they prepared for reentry. All spacecraft systems seemed to be working perfectly.

The spacecraft made a normal landing in central Russia and a recovery helicopter quickly landed along side. When crews opened the hatch, they found the three cosmonauts were still strapped in their couches, all of them dead. Investigation showed a leak had developed in the craft during reentry, and the cabin lost pressure, killing the men almost instantly.

Four years earlier, America had lost three astronauts in the Apollo-One launch pad fire, and the deaths of Gus Grissom, Ed White, and Roger Chaffee had brought critics of the space program out in droves.

Any person associated with high-tech projects, the cutting edge of science, understood and accepted the risks of exploration involved in the advancement of knowledge. But NASA's manned spaceflight programs appeared to be beating the odds, and the agency was very alert to public opinion.

Unknowingly, with Jim Irwin, NASA had sent an astronaut to the moon with coronary artery disease, with a real risk of experiencing "sudden death" anytime during the twelve day mission. Unknowingly, I too carried the same risk with me every day.

In 1971, flight surgeons did not have the tools that are available today to detect the disease, and if there was a death on the moon, space program critics and fortune tellers would take to the streets screaming, "I told you so."

But on July 30th, 1971 Jim and Dave Scott were on the moon, ready to spend a record three days exploring one of the most scientifically interesting areas on the lunar surface —a narrow valley hemmed in on three sides by the tallest mountains on the moon, and on the fourth by the mile-wide canyon, Hadley Rille.

Emphasizing the scientific nature of their mission, Jim Irwin, Dave Scott, and Al Worden named their Apollo-15 spacecraft Endeavour. Endeavour was the name of the first vessel to sail the seas for science—British Captain James Cook's ship, which explored the Pacific in 1768. The astronauts, all Air Force officers, selected Falcon, the Air Force Academy mascot, as the name for the lunar landing craft.

As Dave Scott and Jim Irwin stepped onto the surface of the moon for the first time, the seventh and eighth men to leave their footprints there, they gazed at the dazzling, incandescent light of the lunar morning and absorbed the stark and lonely beauty of the scene.

"As I stand here on the wonders of the unknown at Hadley, I sort of realize there is a fundamental truth to our nature," Dave Scott said. "Man must explore. And this is exploration at its greatest."

Then he and Jim Irwin turned their attention to a machine the world was waiting to see—the first man-driven vehicle on the moon. As a television camera relayed clear pictures to Earth, they operated cables which slowly lowered the $8 million jeep-like vehicle to the surface. Its hollow, wire-mesh wheels snapped into place, and they assembled seats and other parts and loaded aboard geology tools.

"Man, oh man," cried Scott as the moon buggy bounded over the undulating plain at top speed of about eight miles per hour, dodging craters and rocks. "This is really a sporty driving course. What a Grand Prix this is."

Both were strapped in with belts, and Jim Irwin yipped, "Buckin' bronco!"

In three separate excursions over their three-day lunar surface stay, they drove far and wide around the Hadley-Apennine region, collecting one hundred and seventy-one pounds of geological samples, taking photographs, drilling core samples, and vividly describing the scene for scientists.

As a final task, Scott drove the buggy little more than the length of a football field away from the landing craft and pointed it so the television camera mounted on the hood could give earthlings their first look at a blastoff from the moon. Four hours later, Scott and Jim Irwin fired their ascent engine and on the TV screen Falcon suddenly leaped up like a jack-in-the-box and disappeared from sight in just two seconds.

While Jim and Dave spent three days on the lunar surface, crewmate Al Worden was keeping the Apollo-15 spacecraft "Endeavour" orbiting the moon, waiting for them to return.

As soon as Falcon was back in lunar orbit, the two moon walkers powered up the rendezvous radar and went searching for Al Worden in the mother ship Endeavour.

Al must have been forty to fifty miles away when they

first saw his light, and then they left the dark side of the moon and orbited into sunlight where they could see him getting closer and closer.

When they got within a hundred feet, Jim and Dave slowed the lunar module's closure rate and maneuvered right in front of the Apollo-15.

Al Worden lined the mother ship up with Falcon and then they engaged in high style—a good docking. There was a kind of thud as the two space ships came together.

Jim could hear the docking latches grab, and once the two ships were fully mated, Al opened Endeavour's hatch. Jim and Dave opened Falcon's. "Welcome home," Al said.

A cloud of lunar debris moved toward him. Worden threw up a hand in protest. He had a beautiful clean spacecraft and here were these two guys bringing all this moon dust into his neat home. They tried to keep Falcon's hatch closed while they weren't transferring their collection of moon rocks and scientific samples into the Endeavour.

Jim and Dave wanted a few personal souvenirs so they took the utility lights and other loose parts off the lunar module. They were now behind schedule, and suddenly they found themselves hurrying. They knew they had to jettison Falcon at a certain time so that Mission Control could fire its engine by remote control and crash their faithful lunar landing craft into the surface of the moon.

They were rattled by the time squeeze, but they worked quickly, got their jobs done, and Jim was the last to leave. As lunar module pilot he had to make sure all the switches and controls were in their proper position so the ship's engine could be fired from the ground.

Once he was on board Endeavour, the astronauts went through their undocking procedure after the hatches were confirmed closed with a good seal.

"Apollo-15, Houston. Fifteen seconds to LM jettison. Hope you let her go gently; she was a nice one."

The astronauts felt the separation and they watched as Falcon sat there in space as they backed away. Then the ground sent a signal commanding the engine on and Jim and Dave watched their lunar module fall once again toward the moon's surface. They were hoping they might be able to see it hit, but they couldn't. They were in darkness again, still dressed in their bulky space suits, but with helmets and gloves off.

At the same moment, at the flight surgeon's console in Mission Control, the sensors transmitting readings of Jim Irwin's heart rate were reporting a change in his heart's rhythm. The doctor leaned forward, studying the telemetry lines before him. A cold shudder moved through his body. Trouble. Possible life-threatening trouble.

The flight surgeon keyed his mike, relayed what he was seeing to the Flight Director. Deke Slayton, Chief of the Astronaut Office was in the control room. He was brought in for consultation. Was Jim Irwin about to have a heart attack?

A quarter of a million miles from Mission Control, on board Apollo-15 in orbit around the moon, Jim Irwin was tired, bone tired. He stretched out in the weightlessness of space, and stared at his two crewmates.

"Just let me lie here for a little bit," he told Al and Dave. "I am physically exhausted."

This wasn't like Jim. Regardless of how tired he would get in training, or during the flight up to this point, he never begged off. He never offered an excuse. The irregular heart beats were a sign of his fatigue.

Jim lay there for about ten minutes as Dave and Al were getting their suits off, getting ready for bed while in Mission Control a conference was underway among officials and the best medical minds at their command. It was plain Jim had a bigeminal rhythm. With this condition, the impulse for the heart to contract comes from two different sites, alternating with each other. One impulse originates from the normal site located in the upper portion of the right atrium (sinus node). The alternate impulse originates prematurely and from an abnormal site (ventricles). This rhythm reduces the amount of blood pumped out by the heart as the premature abnormal beat is ineffective. The condition is often caused by severe over-exertion in a person with clogged arteries.

The first question for flight surgeons was what could be done? The answer! Nothing. There was no way of getting help to Jim Irwin. There were no medications on board, only sleeping pills.

"How about him taking one of those?" Deke Slayton asked. "Would that help?"

Could, the doctors agreed. Could make sure he rests.

Suddenly, Deke moved into the CAPCOM console, took the mike. *"Apollo-15, Houston."*

"We're here, boss," Jim answered.

"You guys have had a hard day," Deke said. *"I suggest that all of you take a sleeping pill this evening."*

"We hear you, Deke," Jim said, laughing. "We have had a busy day."

Jim simply thought Deke was joking and he managed to remove himself from his space suit. He didn't bother to tell Dave and Al what Deke had said. They were all tired. They didn't need pills to sleep.

After nine hours of sleep, Apollo-15's astronauts woke up. Jim Irwin felt normal in spite of his heart problem, and they spent the next two days in lunar orbit photographing and chemically charting as much of the moon as possible with a seventeen-million-dollar array of cameras, a laser altimeter, and other scientific instruments. Before heading home, they ejected a seventy-eight-pound satellite carrying devices to send back data for a year on magnetic, electrical, and gravity fields.

On the homeward trek, Al Worden took the farthest-out space walk, moving along handrails on the outside of Endeavour to the rear of the ship to retrieve film cassettes from two cameras which had mapped the moon. The stroll, 200,000 miles from earth, was necessary because the service module which housed the cameras would be jettisoned to burn up before reentry.

As Apollo-15 floated downward above the Pacific, one of its three large parachutes collapsed. But the system was designed so the spaceship could land safely on two chutes. The only complication, and it was minor, was a slightly harder landing for the crew.

An hour later, on the deck of the aircraft carrier Okinawa, Apollo-15's primary recovery ship, officials were relieved to see Jim Irwin's heart was beating with a normal rhythm. The first cardiac arrest in space flight had been avoided, but only by dumb luck, and by the grace of God, say some.

In the future, when astronauts settle down for year-long stays on board America's space station Freedom, and when a squadron of two or three planetary ships head for Mars, a medical doctor will surely be a member of the crew, and he or she will be equipped with all the latest equipment and medications.

The Mars trip is expected to take two or three years and it will most likely be an international journey funded by America, Japan, Russia and European nations.

The flight surgeon selected for the awesome mission must be qualified not only to handle the planetary astronauts' medical needs, but he or she must be trained and prepared to perform all types of general surgery in a weightless environment.

As the script writers say, it will be exciting duty on history's most fantastic voyage.

EIGHT

"Age"

Following the success of the Apollo moon landings, American astronauts used the big spacecraft to visit the country's first space station, Skylab, and set space endurance records.

By July 1975, the last Apollo space ship was on the launch pad, and flew an international "goodwill" mission by docking with a Russian Soyus spacecraft.

The Apollo-Soyus flight was called a "Handshake in Space," and was commanded by veteran astronaut Tom Stafford. Deke Slayton, one of the original Mercury Seven who had been grounded for twelve years by a heart irregularity, was cleared for what would be his only mission.

We members of the Cape Canaveral press corps knew that with the conclusion of the Apollo-Soyus flight, America had willed space to the Soviets and it would be several years before another American manned ship would enter orbit.

The mid 1970s was a time we began concentrating on other assignments, and it was also a time I began to notice those doing reports on television and broadcasting the news on radio were getting younger. The reporters I started out with in the business were falling by the wayside. They were being replaced by capped-teeth beauties from both sexes. If it had not been for the fact I agreed to take less pay, and my reporting was specialized in space, I too would have been looking for work.

It was also a time worries appeared on the health front.

My brother Larry was in his mid fifties and the clock of heredity was right on time. He was having troubles with heart disease and with a stubborn attitude that he could find all the help he needed with a local doctor in our small hometown of Blakely, Georgia.

A few days before Christmas 1975, Larry suffered a heart attack, and I went to Blakely in hopes of being some help.

As I drove around the familiar town square I was reminded of the fact the town hadn't changed since I was a kid. It hadn't grown and it hadn't diminished in size. It was the same.

I parked my car, got out, and stood quietly, studying the green before me. The red-brick county courthouse was there, white-pillared and surrounded by live oaks, cedars and magnolia trees. It stood, as if untouched, since strong backs labored its brick and mortar into final form before the Depression. My eyes searched the acre green, seeing the square spiked with cars parked at odd angles, and through the afternoon shadows from moss-draped trees, I saw people amble across the square, watched them go in and out of stores—some of the same stores that were there when I was a kid.

I crossed the street and walked about the square where the world seemed to glow with peculiar brightness. I stopped before a monument to honor the Confederate dead. The words, chiseled in the memorial's granite flank, read:

LEST WE FORGET THOSE WHO DIED
FOR LOCAL SELF GOVERNMENT

A few feet away a bronze marker mounted in concrete had been set in earth at the base of a tall pine pole, the only Confederate flagstaff still standing in Georgia. A monument to strong-willed farmers armed with only shotguns who, two weeks after the War Between The States, stood off an entire company of marauding Union troops. The soldiers in blue had come with axes to fell the staff, but the farmers were prepared to die for this single surviving symbol of the cause for which they had fought. The Union soldiers decided enough blood had been spilled on piney wood battlefields and they marched away, axes over shoulders, singing "John Brown's body lies a' moldering in its grave." The farmers, hurrahing Dixie, wrapped the flagpole in rags of Confederate uniforms. The bronze marker still reads:

THIS FLAGPOLE FROM WHICH THE STARS AND BARS PROUDLY FLEW IS THE LAST ORIGINAL CONFEDERATE FLAGSTAFF STILL STANDING IN GEORGIA. THE STAL-WART POLE WAS HEWN FROM A LONG LEAF PINE TREE THAT GREW ONE MILE SOUTHWEST OF THIS CITY IN EARLY COUNTY. IT WAS HAULED BY A YOKE OF OXEN INTO BLAKELY AND ERECTED WHERE IT NOW STANDS ON MAY 16TH, 1861.

Oddly heroic, it stands without apology. I wondered what my black friends would think about the flagpole. I could only hope they would understand.

It was this fierce independence, this town's self reliance that I knew so well. It was this same self reliance that was preventing my brother from getting quality medical care.

I slipped behind the wheel of my Monte Carlo, turned the ignition key, backed out, and moved slowly into the street to begin the drive around the square.

The only hospital is located on the Dothan highway, little more than a mile from the square, next door to the county nursing home. Our mother, no longer able to cook and take care of herself, had a room there, just a short walk from the intensive care unit where Larry was recovering from his heart attack.

He was one of the most easy-going persons I knew until about two years before his heart attack, when everything seemed to bother him. My mother couldn't do or say anything right, and his business was driving him bonkers. As the only refrigeration and appliance repair man in the small town, he was in constant demand. He couldn't sit down to dinner without the phone ringing, and when he took the name of his company off the side of his truck, it did no good. Everyone knew him, most had bought their appliances and air conditioners from him anyway, and it was his job to make sure they worked as advertised.

A never-satisfied customer with a new trash compactor had been on his back for a couple of days when Larry had his first heart attack. Doctors in Blakely, or anywhere for that matter, weren't too knowledgeable in 1975 about the effects of worry and hostility on heart disease.

I drove into the hospital parking lot and first went by to say hello to Mom before going to Larry's room.

I stood in the door, my eyes focusing on the heart rhythm pattern on the monitor, my ears equally focusing on the constant *beep, beep, beep* . . .

He didn't see me at first, only felt my hand grab his as I walked to his bedside. "Hi Bud," I smiled. "You taking a vacation?"

"Yep," he grinned, "one I didn't schedule."

"How're you feeling?"

"Oh, I feel awright," he said flatly. "In fact I haven't had much pain."

"How'd you know it was a heart attack?"

"Didn't, at first," he said, turning on his side, bracing himself with an elbow. "I was just so mad, and I didn't feel right, and I just came on here to the hospital."

"The tests said it was a heart attack?"

"Yep, that's what that computer said."

"They have a computer here?"

"Naw," he laughed. "They had to send my EKG off, over the phone."

"Well," I said, sitting on the edge of the bed. "We're gonna' get you fixed up. We'll get you the best people in the business."

He looked surprised. "No need for that," he said. "This doctor here is as good as they come."

"Really?" I stared at him. "I don't want to come off as a snob, Bud, but this doctor, and those in Dothan, or even Albany, are run-of-the-mill. The best in the South are located at the University of Alabama at Birmingham," I added. "They're as good as Cleveland or Houston."

"My man here is just as good," Larry said. "They say he's the best."

"Who is they, Bud?"

"People. People who've had heart attacks."

"Well," I smiled. "That's good to know. You deserve the best."

I stood up, walked to the chair across the room and sat down. There was no cause to agitate Larry. It wasn't the time or the place to worry him. The important thing was for him to recover, of course, and it was important that I be as supportive and understanding as possible.

Later, when he was strong again, I would convince him that the Mayo Clinic wasn't in his neighborhood, and he should go where they specialized in treatment of heart disease. After all, lurking somewhere in the back of my mind, was the realization that the body of my brother lying there in bed was identical to the body I had also inherited. The difference? Thirteen years.

No one loved his brother more than I loved mine, and it was of the utmost importance that we did everything we could to keep him alive, to ensure he would have many more years with us. I also knew by getting him the best, by extending his life, I would be laying a blueprint for my future.

I scolded myself for what seemed to be a selfish thought, but heart disease was our inheritance, and the intelligent thing, it seemed to me, was to go out and fight it, to meet it head on—not to sit back and wait for an attack to come in the night, to send us whimpering to our deaths.

I spent a few days with Larry and Mom, and when it was apparent he was recovering quite well, I made plans to return to the Cape to a family Christmas, with a promise to my brother and myself to research and help Larry chart a smart and prudent course of treatment.

The holidays passed and I had some answers. The most up-to-date physicians told me my brother should have a cardiac catheterization—a procedure where catheters are snaked through a major artery in the groin into a person's heart. There a dye is released and photographs are made of the vital coronary arteries' ability to supply the heart with blood.

At first, Larry wouldn't consider it. He was putting all his faith in his local doctor, but as weeks grew into months, he realized he wasn't getting well. Every little pain brought with it fear he could be having another heart attack. I finally convinced him the only way he was ever going to know was by having the people in Birmingham take a look.

In July 1976, Larry was off to the University of Alabama Cardiac Center in Birmingham and we were all pleased— pleased, that is, until I learned he was checking into the Veteran Administration's hospital across the street.

Friends of mine in the medical field threw up red flags immediately. "V.A. hospitals are the pits," one doctor told me. "Can't you help him out financially?"

"Of course I could and would if that was necessary," I told him. "But it's not necessary. He has the insurance, even the cash money."

"Well, why in God's name doesn't he stay in the university hospital, with the experienced university staff?"

"Stubborn," I told the doctor, shaking my head. "He rode a tank through Europe for General Patton during World War II, and he thinks he deserves it."

"Well, I'm sure he does," said my doctor friend. "But he deserves the best treatment."

Again, I tried to tell my brother this. Begged him to stay in the Alabama cardiac center. But he didn't. He was wheeled across the street for the cardiac catheterization and the results were frightening. Two of his main coronary arteries were almost closed, barely any blood getting through to the heart. The cardiologist told him he should have an immediate bypass operation.

"Can I go home and think about it?" Larry asked.

"Only if you tell me your Will is in order, and you will sign a legal document exonerating me from any responsibility," the physician said. "You'll probably be dead before you reach your house."

The cardiologist's blunt statement got Larry's attention and he consented to the bypass operation—an operation that went perfectly, and he was wheeled back across the street to the V.A. facility.

Some doctor took Larry off the beta-blocker Inderal before the operation. He had been taking the drug since his heart attack and his heart rate, following the operation, climbed to over two hundred. Seventy-two is normal.

Inderal would have helped keep his heart rate under control, but more importantly, once you are on any of the beta-blocker drugs, it is important that you reduce the dosage very slowly. In some cases, say experts, it is essential for a patient to spend months decreasing the dosage before finally quitting Inderal. If the patient doesn't, the heart increases its rate, and could go into ventricular fibrillation.

My brother's nurse decided to leave early on the second afternoon following his operation, and she filled out her paperwork through 4:00 P.M. Family members left to go shopping, and Larry remained alone, his heart rate over two hundred, PVCs (premature ventricular contractions) being reported on the monitor.

Sometime between 3:20 and 3:50 P.M. local time my brother experienced sudden death. No one knows the time for sure. He was left unattended.

Revival was not possible. He had been dead too long before being found, and when the autopsy was concluded, the report stated the bypass operation was perfect. There was no problem. A racing heart, being left unattended, and the sudden stopping of the beta-blocker Inderal killed Larry Smith Barbree at age fifty-six.

With my grief I felt guilt. I was covering the campaign of Jimmy Carter for President, and had trouble breaking away. I will always feel if I had, and if I had been there, I would not have permitted his heart rate to climb without getting help. I would not have allowed the nurses to leave him unattended. I know I would have known better. The burden of not being there is mine. The decision not to stay in a first-class heart facility was my brother's.

I felt like calling my friend Ron Nessen, who was Press Secretary to President Gerald Ford at the time, to "nuke" that hospital, but the family wouldn't let me. Why, I will never understand. It may have prevented many future unnecessary deaths. But as I said, southwest Georgia people are stubborn. They march to their own drummers. What makes sense to most, doesn't necessarily to them.

We buried my brother. Jimmy Carter was elected President and I became increasingly concerned about my own health. I was most aware that what had happened to Larry would probably happen to me. It was only a question of when. The inheritance of coronary artery disease was a ticking time bomb within my chest, and during my annual physical at the Watson Clinic in Lakeland, Florida, I demanded a treadmill stress test.

"Oh, we don't give them to people your age, Jay," my doctor, John Simmonds, said.

I told him about my brother, about my family history. Immediately he changed his mind. He told me to stop puffing on the cigarette I had in my hand, and he went about setting up the test. My tobacco-punished lungs kept me going for only six minutes on the treadmill when the first indication of coronary artery disease reared its ugly head.

The treadmill test was stopped and I was sent to Gainesville, Florida to a cardiology expert named Howard Ramsey. There I had my first cardiac catheterization, and as I expected, coronary artery disease was already established in my coronary arteries.

Dr. Ramsey didn't feel it had advanced to the point that a bypass operation was necessary. He sent me home with a prescription for the beta-blocker Inderal to keep my blood pressure and heart rate in check.

When I saw my cardiologist, Dr. Sarvanna Rajan, he suggested that in view of my family history I watch my cholesterol by improving my diet and by exercising.

I made the decision to do everything possible to prevent the growth of my heart disease, and I began my exercise program by first walking five to six miles each day. Soon I was into jogging, only short distances at first, but within a year I was running three to five miles a day.

I was proud of myself and I often bored my friends with my devotion to running.

"You people who jog are snobs about it," mutual friend Harold Williams told me and Astronaut Deke Slayton. "If you gotta' do it, keep it to yourself."

"Jealousy," Deke and I said, and I was finally feeling

good about my health. I felt I was doing okay, and the filthy tobacco habit fell by the wayside.

I spent the last half of the 1970s decade covering President Jimmy Carter's vacations and "down home" holidays, and approached the 1980s confident, in spite of the fact that younger reporters were now getting choice assignments. I consoled myself, the flights of the space shuttles was the story for the 1980s, and I had covered them. I was satisfied with my small slice of the pie.

The first twenty-five missions went by so fast, and so successfully, during the first half of the '80s, that the public was again becoming disinterested in the flights.

NASA's *can do* attitude and safety record had people regarding the space shuttle missions as being safe as flying an airliner, and the fact that U. S. Senator Jake Garn was permitted to go into orbit didn't help discredit that belief.

As chairman of the Senate subcommittee that oversaw NASA's budget, the Senator sometimes joked during hearings that he would not vote for the space agency's budget if he did not get to ride on a space shuttle. When NASA finally said okay, critics accused Garn of using his political clout to make the ultimate congressional junket. But the Utah Republican, a former Navy Pilot, brushed off the carping and, after four months of training, he rode the shuttle Discovery into orbit on April 12th, 1985.

To make himself useful on the journey, Garn volunteered to be a medical guinea pig to help doctors better understand space sickness, which has afflicted about half of shuttle fliers as they adapted to weightlessness.

Well, Senator Jake Garn turned out to be a perfect subject. He was sick the whole flight and when he appeared on TV from space, he had to be held upright by velcro which stuck his body to a wall of Discovery's crew cabin. Since that day, shuttles fly with the "Memorial Jake Garn Wall" for all those who need a barf bag.

Congressman Bill Nelson, Senator Garn's counterpart in the House of Representatives, was also invited to make a shuttle space flight, and he did so without getting sick.

Next, America's first "citizen in space" was ready to ride. For years, we members of the news media had been told that the first citizen would be a journalist, but, because of a campaign promise made by President Reagan to teachers' organizations and unions, the first "citizen in space" would now be a teacher. A Journalist would follow next.

Sharon Christa McAuliffe, a thirty-seven-year-old social sciences teacher from Concord, New Hampshire was selected over 11,000 other applicants; and to be the first Journalist-In-Space, 1,705 filled out applications.

The applications were very specific, very structured, and long. I applied.

Filling out the application was a tedious process with the most demanding portion being the essays.

The applications were, in reality, traps for those who would pay short shrift to the document, because the application was to be used as the first means of reducing the field of applicants to a total of 100.

Not only did I have my fears about coronary artery disease to worry about, again I found myself competing with younger journalists, and I decided if I was going to try to get the assignment in space, I would have to make a dedicated and serious effort.

I read the application over and over, searching for every meaning and intent behind every word, and after writing the two essays, I put them away for a couple of days to give them a chance to breathe.

I polished the essays over and over, and when the application hit the mail, I was satisfied I had done everything possible to be selected as one of the one hundred semi-finalists.

What worried me was the big names I was up against. Tom Brokaw, Sam Donaldson, Walter Cronkite, Jim Hartz, and hundreds of more better known journalists. But when the one hundred were announced, I was one, and I was pleased to learn we had been judged by professors from university journalism schools on our applications, not our stardom.

My friend and colleague Robert Bazell, NBC's Science Editor, also made the one hundred, but our friend Tom Brokaw missed. I would later learn none of the current network anchors were really considered, because there was an unwritten understanding that if one network anchor had been selected over the other, the other nets would pay little notice to the project.

During that time, my contract was coming up for renewal and being in the Journalist-in-Space contest helped. Once again my career was in high gear. I was jogging three to five miles a day and I felt good. I was sure I was ready to ride a shuttle into orbit, and on January 27th, 1986, one day before the shuttle Challenger would lift off with teacher Christa McAuliffe, the first "citizen in space," I signed my new contract with NBC News.

All of us in the Journalist-in-Space Project were wishing we were the one who was taking the first citizen ride, but Christa was a real champion. After interviewing her I understood easily why she was selected. She was the best the country had to offer, and, I knew, the journalist's day would come.

For me, things were definitely looking up.

NINE

"Challenger"

Hugh Harris stared at the numbers before him. Green and flickering with each passing second of the countdown; the television monitors showing him every detail of the shuttle Challenger sitting on its launch pad. He wasn't completely comfortable with the electronics and he often peered out the huge glass window, trusting his own eyes to make sure everything was in its place.

Hugh had been the "Voice of Launch Control" for most of the previous twenty-four space shuttle flights, plus hundreds of unmanned rocket launches, and as Chief of Information for the Kennedy Space Center, he was comfortable with the familiar routine in Launch Control.

This was the fifth launch attempt for this mission for Challenger, and the only thing that was different was Christa McAuliffe was on board.

McAuliffe was seated below the flight deck and was ready to become America's first "citizen in space." But there were those among the astronaut corps that were not ready to see that. Some had protested permitting anyone to fly into orbit except astronauts. They wanted to keep space flight in the sole possession of an elite pilot, engineer, and science corps. These astronauts had to be constantly reminded they were riding a vehicle bought and paid for by American taxpayers and it belonged to all Americans.

When Americans opened the West and other frontiers,

the tough scouts with an instinct for survival cut the trails, but they were followed by the people, by teachers, doctors, lawyers, farmers, blacksmiths, every profession needed along with the families necessary for support.

Sharon Christa McAuliffe was the first of the people, the first citizen willing to risk her life so that she could perform in a classroom from space, and when she boarded Challenger, a member of the closeout crew presented the teacher with an apple. Millions of school children were waiting eagerly to participate in lessons she planned to teach from orbit.

The other crew members were Crew Commander Francis R. "Dick" Scobee, a self-educated tough test pilot who had fought his way up from the enlisted ranks to become one of the country's best; pilot Michael J. Smith; Ellison S. Onizuka, Ronald E. McNair, Judith A. Resnik, and Gregory B. Jarvis, a Hughes Aircraft Company satellite engineer who twice was bumped from earlier flights, those that carried Senator Jake Garn and Congressman Bill Nelson.

The countdown moved through T-minus two minutes and Commander Dick Scobee grinned inside his locked helmet visor, "Welcome to space, guys."

Inside launch control the last-moment events kept rolling from the lips of Hugh Harris, through his microphone, and to the hundreds of broadcast and press outlets receiving the NASA Select service.

"T-minus ten, nine, eight, seven, six, we have main engine start. . . ."

*I*gnition began in a swift rippling fashion, a savage fire birth tearing at the eyes of thousands of onlookers, and a blizzard fell, a swirling ice storm shaken from the flanks of Challenger's ten-story-tall external tank.

Seconds passed, the main engines screaming, waiting for the computers to sense all three were running properly, had built up lift-off thrust, and a signal was sent to ignite and free the two giant boosters.

Flame raged, kicked out two large pillows of fire and

steam as the boosters ignited, slammed their six million pounds of thrust into thousands of gallons of water and into launch pad 39B, lifting off in an insanity of fire, fiercer, then brighter.

"

. . . four, three, two, one, and lift off, lift off of the twenty-fifth space shuttle mission and it has cleared the tower."

*I**nside Challenger's crew cabin at ignition of the three main engines, Crew Commander Scobee shouted, "There they go, guys."*

"Alllll riiiight!" yelled Judy Resnik.

"Three at a hundred," reported Scobee.

"Alllll riiiight!" screamed Judy again.

"Here we go," laughed pilot Mike Smith, and Challenger leaped off its pad, thundering skyward on a 700 foot tail of fire and billowing smoke from the giant solid boosters.

The rocket ship lifted higher and flame splashed madly, went screaming in all directions, a howling fire broom sweeping away everything before it.

The astronauts' families stood in the shadow of the giant Vehicle Assembly Building, more than three miles away, and before the sound reached them the earth trembled, then shook. The air danced before their eyes as shock waves raced across the palmetto and scrub brush, vibrated their bones and jiggled their eyes.

Mouths open, shouting, but no one hearing the words as the roar inundated them and lightning bolts of raw thunder exploded in their midst.

They reached out, eyes shining, sought each others' hands, and held each other tightly.

*Something sinister occurred when the solid fuel rockets ig-
nited. Unseen by anyone, a large puff of black smoke spat
forth from the lower joint on the right booster as the giant
rocket rotated every so slightly, opening a tiny gap. The primary O-ring seal was too cold to seat and to seal immediately.
The night before the temperature had dipped into the twen-
ties, an unusual freeze for Cape Canaveral, and the cold-stiff-
ened putty in the joint collapsed. Hot gases with a temperature of nearly 6,000 degrees rushed past an area of the
primary seal, and because of the joint rotation, the second
O-ring was not in its sealed position and the gases blasted
past.*

*The puffs of black smoke continued for two and one-half
seconds, then stopped when aluminum oxides from the burning fuel miraculously plugged the leaks in the joint before the
flame could escape.*

*Unaware they were in mortal danger, the astronauts
were excited as Challenger climbed higher and higher.*

*"Go you mother!" pilot Mike Smith shouted as Chal-
lenger rolled into its proper flight path.*

*"LVLH," reported Judy Resnik, reminding the pilots of a
cockpit switch change.*

"Ohhhhkaaaay," Dick Scobee grinned.

The sound and fury rushed swiftly to the press site. Less
than one hundred journalists who regularly covered the
shuttle launches saw Challenger break free, saw red become
orange as a dazzling golden fire savaged the shuttle launch
mesa.

No matter how many of these launches you had seen,
no matter how many times you had felt the body-shaking
impact, heard the thunderous outpouring of sonic violence,
you never felt at ease, never took man's flights into orbit for
granted.

Reuters' veteran space reporter Mary Bubb sat in the
press site's bleachers, watching Challenger thunder skyward.
She groped for the hand of the reporter sitting beside her.

"I'm afraid," the ailing reporter said, her voice barely audible over the roar. "I'm afraid for them."

*S*hear *winds up to 84 miles per hour, some of the highest ever for a shuttle flight, struck Challenger as it passed through Max Q—maximum aerodynamic stress—prompting pilot Mike Smith to remark, "Looks like we've got a lotta' wind here today."*

"Yeah," Scobee acknowledged, "It's a little hard to see out my window."

When the winds hit the right booster rocket, they jarred loose the aluminum oxides that had sealed the lower joint. There was now nothing to hold back the fire. A tongue of flame burst through the joint opening, creating a blowtorch at the 58-second mark in the flight.

"Okay, we're throttling down," Dick Scobee said as he began reducing the power of the main engines from 104 percent to 94 percent to 65 percent, holding down the energy while the shuttle knifed its way through the high winds and maximum aerodynamic stress. Then, he restored full power, throttling back up to full thrust on the engines.

"Feel the mother go," Mike Smith yelled.

"Wooooohooooo," another crew member shouted.

"35,000 going through one point five," Smith reported.

"Reading 486 on mine," Scobee told his pilot.

Smith acknowledged the routine airspeed check. "Yep that's what I've got too."

Scobee listened as Mission Control reported his engines were running fine at full throttle again—everything was "GO."

"Roger, go at throttle up," Dick Scobee reported in the matter-of-fact language of the seasoned test pilot.

But what Dick Scobee and the rest of his crew did not know was that the tongue of flame that had burst through the lower field-joint-splice on the right booster, had burned through and collapsed the lower half of the external fuel tank, where the liquid hydrogen that fed the main engines was stored. When the lower strut that attached the booster to

*the tank broke away, the rocket swiveled on its upper strut
and its nose crashed into the top of the tank, freeing liquid
oxygen to mix with the hydrogen and create the massive fireball seen by spectators, and that would be seen by television
viewers for weeks to come.*

Inside Mission Control Nasa commentator Steve Nesbitt
was following the script before him, reporting the engines
were now burning at 104 percent, full thrust. He took his
eyes away from the monitors, the giant television screen on
the wall in the control center, and continued to read his prepared notes.

"One minute and fifteen seconds, velocity 2900 feet per
second, altitude nine nautical miles, down range distance
seven nautical miles."

A nearby flight controller waved at him, pointed toward
the screen. He stared disbelieving at the expanding fire
cloud, the twisting smoke trails painted across the sky by the
boosters, the chunks of fiery debris raining toward the Atlantic.

Nesbitt slumped in his seat. He felt like he had been run
over, had a house dropped on him, and he sat there while he
felt what seem to be his blood draining from his body.

He shook off the helpless feeling and keyed his mike.
"Flight controllers here are looking very carefully at the situation. Obviously a major malfunction."

He slumped back in his chair. Caught his breath. Listened to the Flight Director's loop. "We have no down link,"
he continued. "We have a report from the flight dynamics
officer that the vehicle has exploded. The Flight Director con-
firms that, uh, we're looking at, uh, checking with the recovery forces to see what can be done at this point."

*At the point of explosion, pilot Mike Smith was suddenly
aware something awful was happening. He uttered the final
words preserved on a spacecraft recorder, "Uh Oh!"*

After that loss of all data, experts think the forces on Challenger at breakup were probably too low to cause death or serious injury to the crew but were sufficient to separate the crew compartment from the forward fuselage, cargo bay, nose cone, and the forward reaction control compartment— the thruster rockets that control the shuttle's position.

The seven astronauts may have remained conscious for a few seconds or longer as the ship broke up at 48,000 feet. Challenger then soared to its peak altitude of 65,000 feet before plummeting through an arc that took it two and three-quarter minutes to impact the Atlantic.

Hugh Harris sat stunned in Launch Control, staring through the big window, still not convinced he was looking at that much fire and destruction in the deep blue sky.

What made it so unbelievable was he knew how much the launch team and all the workers at the space center cared. He sat there wondering how it could have happened.

Quickly, he dismissed the sentiment, promising himself he would grieve later in private. Now was the time to move professionally.

First, he called the news center. "Don't let anyone have the video tapes. We need them for those networks and stations not here. Hold onto those tapes," he ordered, turning around to speak with Jesse Moore, the highest ranking NASA executive in the center.

Moore was NASA's Associate Administrator for Space Flight, and Hugh explained he would have to say something to the public, speak to the news media as soon as possible.

The stunned official stood there, not quite sure what he and his management team should first do.

In The First, F.A. Bank on Route A1A in Cocoa Beach, Jo Barbree and her colleagues stood watching debris from the destruction of Challenger fall toward the ocean. No one had a clear understanding what was happening, but Jo had been around launches long enough, she knew something was terribly wrong.

A customer drove into the drive in window and she went to wait on her. The radio was blaring in the customer's car, and an uninformed news type was telling the world how the astronauts had been ordered to return and land at the shuttle landing strip on the Cape.

"I don't think so," Jo said quietly.

A well-known astronaut was in a bed other than his wife's, and his woman friend shook him anxiously. They had made love most of the night and sleeping until noon seemed the thing to do.

She prodded him again. "Honey, please get up."

"What for?" he questioned.

"There's something funny, a strange noise," she said. "I think they launched the shuttle."

"Whatta' you mean, funny?" he questioned her again, placing his face in the hollow of her neck, biting gently, tasting her salty perspiration.

"Honey, will you get up and look for God's sake?"

He rolled onto his back with a grunt, sat up, and placed his feet on the floor. There was a low rumble washing through the walls of the condo and he forced himself to his feet, walked to the window and saw the sky.

"Mother of God," he said, quietly.

Harry Kolcum, veteran editor of the magazine Aviation Week, stood in front of the press site's bleachers, staring at something he knew he would think about, and dream about, for the rest of his life. He didn't really want to call the office, talk to anyone about what had just happened, but he turned and started walking toward his phone in the press dome.

Reuter's Mary Bubb left the stands with that terrible image in her mind. She knew she would see Challenger exploding in her mind forever.

Along the way, she heard another reporter ask, "Did you see the faces? The faces, I'll never forget the faces."

Inside the United Press International wire service trailer, aerospace reporter Bill Harwood was madly typing copy into his computer terminal, sending the story out over the wire as quickly as possible when suddenly he stopped. "Dammit!" he screamed. "They're dead. They're all *dead.*"

Next door to UPI, veteran aerospace writer Howard Benedict was doing the same thing for the Associated Press—getting the word out as quickly as possible. But Benedict was dictating his story over the phone to the wire service's New York desk. His first paragraph was already on all wires as a bulletin, and he was dictating his second paragraph: "There was no immediate indication on the fate of the crew, but it appeared that nobody could have survived that fireball in the sky."

Inside all the broadcast studios on the press site hill—the CBS building, the ABC building, the CNN trailer, our own NBC building—all networks were live.

Tom Brokaw was in Washington on other business, but he quickly made his way to the NBC Washington Studios to anchor the Challenger disaster coverage.

In the TV studio at the Cape producer Kelly Rickenbacher and his skeleton crew had correspondent Steve Delaney on the air. Because shuttle launches had become so routine, only CNN was on the air live with the blowup, and the others were there in the event of an emergency.

It was Steve Delaney's first trip to the Cape in years and I wished him luck. I had the NBC radio network to worry about.

A strange *feeling,* a feeling of impending disaster I have never been able to understand or explain, swept over me just moments before Challenger exploded.

Because of it, I dialed the New York desk, received a circuit reorder. I dialed again, luckily ahead of all the calls that would soon flood the Cape's phone system, making getting an available telephone line impossible.

The desk picked up just as Challenger exploded, and I said firmly to Jim Wilson, the senior producer, "Don't hang up this line, Jim. We'll never be able to get another out of here."

"Why is that, Jay?"

"We've had a disaster."

"You've had what?"

"Do you have NASA Select up on a monitor?"

"Yeah, we sure do," he said, turning. "Oh my God, Jay, what is it?"

"It's exploded, Jim, but wait," I said, "I wanta' see if Challenger is okay."

I pulled the phone down by my side, searched the destruction in the sky above me, kept looking for Challenger, kept hoping it would reappear out of that growing fireball, hoping it would glide to a pancake landing on the Atlantic, possibly make a return to the shuttle landing strip only a couple of miles away. But it didn't.

I held my emotions in check, lifted the phone to my quivering lips and said, "First, Jim, tell Farley to send help. I can't cover this by myself."

"Understand," he said.

"Now, let's hit the air with a hotline."

Jim Wilson sprung into action. He's one of the best NBC News has, and he called the normally, unflappable Cameron Swayzee into the studio to anchor the hotline bulletin.

A nervous, out-of-breath Cameron Swayzee spoke into the studio microphone: "This is an NBC News Hotline Report. This is correspondent Cameron Swayzee at NBC News Headquarters in New York.

"There has been a major malfunction problem with the
space shuttle Challenger which moments ago lifted off from
Cape Canaveral. Details are not certain yet, but let's go to
Cape Canaveral and try to bring in correspondent Jay Barbree who's standing by.

"Jay, are you there, and what can you tell us?"

Inside, I was telling myself to be calm, be professional.
Feelings would have to wait. "Cameron, we're looking at a
disaster in the blue skies above this spaceport. A major disaster. The space shuttle Challenger, only a minute or so after
lift off, exploded. We have nothing but fire and debris in the
sky . . ."

I didn't say so on the air, but it was obvious the astronauts had died in that *Hell* above me. In journalism, in reporting death, you wait. Wait until there's official confirmation. That confirmation would come, for me, a couple of
hours later when flags around the space center were lowered
to half staff. That's when I reported the crew had been lost.
In the first post-Challenger news conference an hour later,
NASA Associate Administrator Jesse Moore confirmed it.

Meanwhile, during the first hours following the disaster, thousands of journalists were running for planes,
headed for the Cape, and NBC News was no exception. We
were moving troops in from our Miami Bureau as well as
New York, and in the New York control center they were
madly searching for material, new things to say, new information about the blowup, but NASA had shut up, no information was coming from the agency.

Why? It was simply in chaos. No real plans for such a
disaster was in place. There had even been one report to
officials that Challenger had been brought down with a single bullet from a high-powered rifle.

All video tapes, pictures, films of the launch were being
confiscated. Decisions just simply were not being made.
Many of the old hands that had nursed NASA's space program from its infancy had been forced into retirement by a
new breed of executives skilled in politics. They were not
hands-on engineers. None of them could make a rocket or
spacecraft fly. They were politicians and they had simply
flown south with their carpet bags and wormed their way

into one of the most successful programs in the country. They now had one major problem. What did they do now? Who could they blame this on? How could they protect their own asses?

But below this top rung of politicians were men and women who knew what to do, and they got busy. Level two and three management people were off and running, trying to pick up the pieces from a horrible decision that had violated one simple rule that had been in place since Project Mercury. *You don't take chances with astronauts' lives!*

As the bucket ran lower and lower on water, NBC TV decided they needed me on with Tom Brokaw. They needed to reach back into the history of the space program, they needed to know what my sources were telling me.

An out-of-breath Kelly Rickenbacher came bursting into the radio studio. "They want you on TV," he said.

I stared at him. "I'm on radio, Kelly, I can't leave my post."

The producer stared at me. "But they want you on TV," he protested.

"Let me check with my desk," I told him, turning to pick up the open line.

"Hell no, you won't go on TV," Jim Farley screamed down the phone line. "You're our man, we need you there."

Jim Farley was Vice President of Radio Network News, and he went on to tell me he would take the heat for his decision. I explained this to Kelly, and he left, only to return in a few minutes to tell me the President of NBC News, Larry Grossman, wanted me on TV. I told the radio desk that I wasn't going to disobey the President, and soon I was running back and forth between Radio and Television news.

That evening, NBC News executives decided I had best devote my efforts to investigating the accident, trying to learn what had gone wrong. They sent in all the help we could use, and the next morning, I hit the ground running.

The smartest thing New York did was to send Don Browne, the Director of the Miami Bureau, to take charge. Don is a real heavy-weight, a get-things-done kind of man; a man who treats every person, black, white, Hispanic, equally. He harnesses abilities, frees talent to produce the best possible product for NBC News. He's not afraid to step on a few toes when necessary. He doesn't devote ninety percent of his time to covering his rear, shifting blame elsewhere. What you see is what you get, and I was glad to see him there. I knew we were gonna' kick some competitors' asses.

"Jay," he said in a no-nonsense tone. "You're the best chance we have of breaking this story."

"Yes sir."

"I don't want you getting involved in anything else."

"Yes sir."

"We'll handle the running news," he said, his tone still firm. "We'll cover the NASA briefings, the handouts, the stuff everybody's getting."

"I understand, Don."

"You get us what NASA's not telling us."

"I gotta' go see some people, make some calls."

"You do whatever it takes. You're on your own. Get back to me with whatever you learn."

"Yes sir," I said, going out the trailer door, anxious to get started.

I locked myself in my office and started making phone calls, talking with the grunts that turned the wrenches on the launch pad as well as supervisors and management types. I kept getting the same opinion. No fact. Nothing for sure. But opinion.

"It had to be one of the main engines," one management type told me (I can't use names, violate confidentiality). "We're really pushing the state of the art with those babies. You know about the explosions we had on the test stands."

"Haven't you been worried about a fan letting go? Ripping everything to pieces?" I asked.

"That's right. That's what I believed happened."

I kept getting the same story from everyone until one engineer made an off-hand comment about a concern raised the day before the launch by a small group of Morton Thiokol engineers in Brigham City, Utah.

Thiokol built the solid rocket boosters for the space shuttle, and after further investigation, I learned that the engineers were concerned about earlier problems with the joints between booster segments. They decided to alert management at NASA's Marshall Space Flight Center in Alabama. Marshall oversees the booster's design and production, and the group decided to tell management that the cold weather could seriously affect those joints.

Their concern was with the synthetic rubber O-rings designed to seal the joints and prevent hot gases and flames from escaping. On several shuttle flights, the primary O-ring had suffered severe hot gas erosion, and in a few instances minor erosion was found on the secondary O-ring seals. The lower the outdoor temperature, the greater the erosion, with fifty-three degrees the lowest temperature to that time.

I learned that on August 19, 1985, Marshall and Thiokol officials briefed NASA headquarters for the first time on the history and potential of the O-ring problem. They had not recommended halting flights, saying that continuing to fly was an acceptable risk while the joints were being redesigned.

Acceptable risk? What the hell ever happened to the spirit of Mercury, Gemini, Apollo? No risk is acceptable when it comes to protecting the lives of the astronauts.

I called a solid management source in the Marshall office and asked him about the O-ring concern.

"Oh, we had two teleconferences on that Monday," he said. "It was decided that wouldn't be a problem. Everybody signed off on it. We agreed we should fly."

"You don't think the O-rings was the problem?"

"Naw," he assured me. "It was one of the engines."

"You know that for sure?"

"No, not yet, but we're looking," he said. "Something came loose, something let go, and we lost a crew."

"A fan?"

"Could be," he agreed, but quickly added, "Don't go with that yet, Jay. That's what we think it is. I'll let you know when we've got something."

I thanked my management friend at Marshall and decided to take a break, go to the press dome, see if I could get a moment with my friend Hugh Harris.

I knew NASA's Chief of Information wouldn't tell me anything he wouldn't tell the rest of the press, but I also knew if I let him know what I knew, sometimes I could read his reaction, I could tell if I really was on to something.

"Jay, do you really want to know what happened?" Hugh asked, smiling.

"Sure, of course," I said eagerly, realizing I was being reeled in.

"The truth is, Jay," Hugh's tone became serious. "We don't know what happened. We simply don't know anything yet."

"I'm hearing the engines are the main suspect."

"Possibly," Hugh said soberly. "But the engines are only one of thousands of possibilities."

"The bottom line is no one knows."

"Right," Hugh said. "A lot of rumors, but nothing concrete."

I nodded I understood, and said, "Hugh, we're friends, and I sincerely would never asked you to tell me anything that would affect your position with NASA."

He nodded he understood and said, "Now let's have the *but!*"

I laughed. "The but is, I'm gonna' be talking to a lot of people, and if I get something I feel is concrete, could I run it by you?"

"Sure," he said, "but this is my *but*, I may not know if what you have is correct or not."

"I understand."

"If I can," he smiled. "I'll try to keep you from getting burned."

I jumped up and kicked my heels. "How could anyone asked for more?"

I returned to my office feeling I knew everything that was known at the moment, but I also knew the reason for Challenger's fate could be discovered at any moment.

Redneck One! The sudden awareness of where I should go hit me in the emptiness between my ears. Redneck One! Sam Beddingfield, the engineer who came here with the Mercury Seven Astronauts, the man who until a couple of weeks ago had been Deputy Director of Shuttle Projects Management—whose job had been eliminated by those carpet baggers that had wormed their way to the top, and had gotten rid of much of manned spaceflight experience. Sam Beddingfield, who had been called a redneck, as I had, by some who feel they are possessed with all the morals and justice in the world.

Hell, Sam and I knew we weren't bigots. We knew we were talking to bigots. And we simply dubbed each other Redneck One, and Redneck Two, and pretty soon we were being called the names with affection, even by our black friends.

I grabbed the phone, listened to the rings. "Hello."

"Redneck One?"

"Hey, there, Redneck Two, what's up."

"Not the Challenger," I said soberly.

"Yeah," Sam said quietly, quickly adding, "Those idiots say they're gonna' fly twenty-four missions a year with half the man power."

"When donkeys fly," I said.

"I bet that's a Chinese fire drill out there today," he said. "The whole fourth floor running around, pointing fingers, protecting their asses."

"Yeah, there's enough blame to go around. They can point some of it in my direction."

"How's that?"

"Hell, Sam," I said. "I should've known what was going on, what caused those guys to lose their lives."

"Why you, Jay?"

"It's my job, buddy. I'm paid to know what's going on here."

"Okay," he said quietly. "Let's say you knew what was going on, knew the danger the astronauts were in, do you think you could have gotten anyone to listen?"

"Maybe," I said. "Maybe not, just like hunter-killer satellites."

"What?"

"The Soviets' hunter-killer satellites," I explained. "I've been reporting on them for more than two years and the other day there was a story in the New York Times about them."

"And?"

"And you know what happened?"

"No."

"The New York desk called me all excited and asked me if I knew anything about hunter-killer satellites."

Sam laughed. "Suddenly, it was news, huh?"

"You got it," I said, adding, "But *the* story now is what caused the Challenger blowup. Can you help me?"

"Sure," Sam said, "but I don't think they know anything yet."

"I think you're right, but," I added, "they're gonna', and when they do I need to know it."

"Hell, I'm retired, Redneck Two, but I don't have anything better to do," he said, excitement in his voice. "I think it's time I visited my old office."

For the next twenty-four-hours Sam Beddingfield parked himself in the executive offices at NASA headquarters, visiting old friends, listening to everything being learned about the accident.

In the middle of the afternoon, Thursday, January 30th, 1986, two days after Challenger exploded nine miles above its launch pad, Sam Beddingfield called me.

"Redneck Two?"

"Yep, this is Two, is that you, Number One?"

"I've got it."

"The cause of the failure?"

"A rupture in a field joint splice."

"An O-ring leak?"

"Right."

"That's it, for sure?"

"For sure."

"They have pictures."

"Whatta' you mean?"

"Pictures of the leak, a flame blowing out of the sucker like a blow torch."

"What did it do, burn into the tank?"

"Yep," he said. "They think it burned through the insulation and everything blew."

"Where did these pictures come from?"

"Film cameras on the north side."

"Away from us?"

"Right."

"We can't see it on our launch tape?"

"No way."

"Can you get your hands on those pictures?"

"No way," he laughed. "You trying to get me shot?"

"No way, Number One."

I asked Sam to educate me on the booster segments, on their joints called "Field Joint Splices," how they were stacked here at the launch site, and once I felt comfortable I had what I should know nailed down, I thanked him, and moved to confirm with a second source.

I called my management friend at the Marshall Space Flight Center office and he confirmed. The warning by the Thiokol engineers should have been heeded.

I looked at my watch. It was 4:00 P.M., more than two and a half hours before Tom Brokaw's Nightly News aired. Damn, I thought, should I go with it now, before someone else breaks it?

I left my office and went into the trailer to see Don Browne. He sat talking on the phone, in what appeared would be a never-ending conversation. Agitated I held a finger before his eyes.

Annoyed he looked up. "Just a minute, Jay."

"Now," I said, "get rid of whoever you're talking to."

He stared at me irritated by the interruption, but then scanning my face he realized I had something important to communicate. "I'll call you back later."

"I got it."

"Got what?"

"The story, the cause of the blowup, dammit."

He took a deep breath, "Let's go somewhere and talk."

We went outside and quickly I laid it out for him. "Let's go back to your office and call New York." he said grimly. Don got Executive Vice President of News John Lane on the phone along with Vice President Joe Angotti. We filled them in.

"Who are your sources, Jay?" John Lane asked.

I looked at Don. I couldn't believe the question. "With all due respect, Mr. Lane," I said. "I don't reveal my sources."

"Well," he said, "we have a policy, we have to know who

the sources are before we put something of this magnitude on the air."

"Mr. Lane," I said firmly. "I do not reveal my sources. Now, you've asked me to investigate this accident, to find the cause, and I have done that." I paused for a moment before continuing. "I have been with this company for nearly twenty-eight years. I have broken my share of exclusives in the past. You have my reputation. If that's not good enough, I suggest you don't carry the story. I'll break it on the Radio Network."

"No," he said, "we want the story, but we have to be sure."

"Dammit, John, I'm sure," Don Browne said. "Jay, has the best sources here. He's proved it time and again. Now, let's get the Nightly people on the phone and let's break it."

I put the phone down. "You argue it out with them," I said. "I wanta' see Hugh."

"Good idea," Don said. "Hurry back."

I went to Hugh Harris' office, got him alone for a moment and laid the whole story in his lap. He was stunned. He hadn't heard a word about it. He was no help, but he was glad to hear what I knew.

I left the dome just in time to see a high-ranking NASA official pulling out of a parking spot, heading back to head-quarters.

I ran to the car, put my hands on the driver's door, told the official what I knew.

He sat there for a moment, starring at the wheel. "You've got it," he said, still staring straight ahead.

"Thank you."

He turned to face me. "I'm on my way to my office now to look at the pictures."

I ran back to my office where Don Browne was still on the the phone with New York. "Hold on," he said, "Jay's back."

"I've just confirmed it with a third source," I said. "If TV doesn't want it, I'm sure Jim Farley does."

"No," Don said. "Nightly is going with it, but we have a problem."

"What?"

"They want Bob Bazell to do the story and quote you."

"Won't be the first time I've been big-footed," I laughed. "Whatever they want. The paycheck's the same."

"Bullshit," Don said. "It's your story. You should do it. Bob's doing another package."

"Whatever," I said. "Let's just get the story on the air. I know Howard Benedict won't be far behind."

"The AP man?"

"Right. He's got good sources too."

Bob Bazell was brought in and the NBC Science Editor agreed with Don Browne. He too felt I should do the story, break it by doing live cross-talk with Tom Brokaw.

Bob and I have always gotten along. He's a fair man, and I left the trailer, left Don Browne to argue with New York and I went in search of a shuttle model. If I was going to demonstrate for Brokaw what went wrong, then I would need a model.

Moving quickly I got Bruce Hall of CBS, a friend and a top-notched journalist, to lend me his.

Don Browne won the argument and that night I broke the story, the biggest of my journalistic life on Tom Brokaw's Nightly News live, and I did it with the New York Times' reporter standing below my position, taking notes.

Breaking the story got me a write-up in the Times, in the Washington Post, in Newsweek, in Time, Inc., and on all the wire services. Two months later I was selected as one of the finalists in the Journalist-in-Space Project.

We applicants had to go before a selection board made up of six journalism professors and five peers, and were questioned by a live TV interviewer, and when it was over, there were eight of us left in the southeast—five in the Washington press corps, two in Florida, and one in Virginia.

Then I settled down for the long haul, the months of covering NASA's recovery from the Challenger accident, and months of keeping in shape for the Journalist flight.

It was a time of little sleep and many frustrations, and a time that you had to get where you were going with deliberate haste.

Only minutes after Challenger was consumed by that giant explosion, what would become the largest naval search and salvage operation ever undertaken was launched. Six thousand people, fifty-two aircraft, thirty-one ships, three submarines and five robot subs were used.

The real pressure began the day civilian divers discovered Challenger's crew cabin with the astronauts' remains in one hundred feet of water seventeen miles northeast of the Cape. Every news editor in the world wanted to know when and if Challenger's crew had been recovered, if each astronaut had been reclaimed from the sea for internment by the family.

It was a time your best simply wasn't good enough.

TEN

"Heros From The Sea"

The water was murky, swirling from surface winds, keeping the two divers from seeing more than an arm's reach in front of them. They had been diving for days, recovering Challenger's debris scattered across the ocean's floor, and now, on this dive, they were running out of air, only six minutes left in their tanks.

They were about one hundred feet down, moving across the sea's floor when they almost bumped into what appeared first to be a mess. A tangle of wire and metal, nothing that unusual. Nothing they hadn't seen on many dives before.

Then, they saw it. A space suit, full of air, legs floating toward the surface. There's someone in it, diver Terry Bailey thought.

No, that's not right, he admonished himself. Shuttle astronauts don't wear space suits during powered flight. They wear jump suits.

He turned to his partner, Mike McAllister. They just looked at each other and thought, Jackpot. This is what we've been looking for. The crew cabin.

Low on air, the two divers made a quick inspection, marked the location with a buoy and returned to their boat to report the find.

I sat in our radio studio, scanning audio tape, listening for a useable sound bite, something I could use on my overnight reports. Suddenly, Danny Noa burst through the door.

"Jay," the television producer shouted, "Sounds like they've found something."

We both ran out of the building to the edit trailer where we had set up a bank of radio receivers to constantly scan the recovery vessels' ship-to-shore transmissions.

"Base, this is the Preserver, we've found the rudder but no speedbrake," the excited voice said.

"Preserver, this is base. What about the speedbrake?"

"Base, this is Preserver. We can only confirm rudder at this time. No speedbrake."

Danny Noa starred at me. "Whatta' you think it is?"

"Don't know," I said, "It doesn't make sense."

"How's that?"

"The rudder speedbrake is one unit. It should be together," I said, puzzled. "Keep listening, Danny, I'm gonna' make a couple of calls."

I ran back to the radio studio and called a source in NASA security. "There's something going on out there," I said. "They've found the rudder but not the speedbrake."

"Like, Hell," the source said. "The rudder speedbrake has already been recovered. I was there when they brought it in."

"It's something else. It's something big," I said quietly.

"Yeah," my source said. "They're using rudder speedbrake as a code. They know you news guys are listening."

"Uh huh! Can you find out anything?"

"I'll try. You at your press site numbers?"

"Right."

I hung up the phone and rushed back to the edit trailer. Danny and the crew were getting everything on paper as well as on tape. I motion him to the side.

"It's not the rudder," I whispered. "The rudder speedbrake has already been recovered. It's gotta' be something big. Let's keep it just between us."

"You think it could be the crew compartment, the astronauts?"

"That's what I'm thinking," I said. "I've never heard them get this excited before."

Danny nodded in agreement.

"Let's keep it quiet, just between us. I don't want it spread over the press mound."

"Right."

"I'm going to shake a few bushes. See what I can find out," I said, going out of the trailer door.

I knew Danny and the Miami crew would stay with it, keep it quiet, and, most importantly, I knew Danny Noa wouldn't be calling the desk and producers in New York prematurely. He wouldn't be trying to "suck up," trying to make himself look good like some I have worked with. He was a solid professional, the story comes first type, and I felt very comfortable working with him. It was like wearing worn and proven clothing. Danny Noa and his Miami crew fit just right.

I fired up my Chevy Van, shifted it in gear, and quickly headed for Port Canaveral. A couple of well-placed Navy sources, contacts you didn't dare speak to over monitored phones, were my best hope.

At sea with the recovery ships, Astronaut Jim Bagian was disgusted with himself. Weeks before Astronauts Robert Crippen and Bob Overmyer had set up the code name "rudder speedbrake" in the event the crew cabin and the astronauts were found. Rudder simply meant the crew compartment. Speedbrake meant the crew, and with the rudder speedbrake already recovered, then there was no chance there could be a mix-up.

The divers McAllister and Bailey didn't have enough air left in their tanks to go exploring so they could not confirm any of the astronauts' remains were in the wreckage. They could only say with some certainty they had found the crew cabin. This is what Astronaut Bagian was trying to transmit to shore.

The message was typed up and driven with great speed to the Astronauts' Quarters on the Kennedy Space Center where veteran shuttle flyers Robert Crippen and Bob Overmyer were located. They had been put in charge of the recovery of the remains of their colleagues, but upon receipt of the message, they were confused.

Overmyer drove immediately to the radio facilities on the Cape and made contact with Jim Bagian.

Several transmissions later, Bob Overmyer understood what Bagian had been trying to tell them, and he and Robert Crippen boarded a ship in port to plan the recovery of the Challenger Seven's remains.

Luck was with me when I reached Port Canaveral. Both sources were in their facilities and within minutes I had learned what I came for. The crew cabin had been found presumably with the astronauts still inside. I got back in the van, driving across the Bee Line causeway, and headed to the press site.

In front of me a Canadian tourist driving one of the large model Mercedes blocked my path. I slowed and stayed behind the big car until we reached the toll booth. I took the correct change lane and the Mercedes' driver approached the booth.

I came out of the gate and accelerated as quickly as I could, trying to reach the press site in time to feed what I felt was an exclusive to Nightly News. I didn't give the Mercedes another thought until it passed me doing about 90 MPH. My speed was about 60, five-miles-per-hour over the speed limit.

The Mercedes slowed about a mile ahead, and fell in line behind a large tractor-trailer truck.

I still wasn't paying too much attention to the Canadian. My mind was on the story, getting back to the press site and getting it on the air.

The truck and the Mercedes were running about the speed limit, and within a couple of minutes I caught up with them. As we approached an overpass, I was in the process of passing when the Mercedes' driver decided he wouldn't let me. The big car pushed its way back into the passing lane, shoving my van up against the bridge's left railing.

My temper snapped. I wouldn't back off. I held my own,

and the three vehicles reached the top of the bridge running side-by-side.

I slammed the van's accelerator to the floor, and the truck driver couldn't believe what he was seeing. Before the powerful Mercedes could burst away with its speed, I eased my van into the car, locking the big machine between my vehicle and the running board and fender of the truck. Groans were heard and sparks flew from the grinding metal, and the Mercedes' driver looked up at me, a face covered with fright. "We're not playing tag you sonofabitch," I screamed, suddenly feeling the steering wheel grow loose in my hands. The weight of the truck and the big car was over-coming my van's grip of the road, and I backed off.

We reached the foot of the bridge still three-abreast where the Mercedes broke free and sped away, leaving my van and the truck in its wake.

The truck driver continued staring at me, disbelieving. He couldn't seem to manage a word or a gesture.

I pushed the accelerator to the floor and moved in front, and soon I was at the turn off to the space center.

"What a dumb thing to do, Barbree," I yelled at myself. "Why in the hell didn't you back off? Being in the right means very little when you're dead."

I drove toward the press site, my temper cooling. Reason returned to my thoughts and I knew I ought to keep my hostility under control, but I really had no idea, combined with heredity, how deadly such outbreaks of temper were to my chances of living a normal lifetime. I shook such moral-istic thoughts off and focused on the story I had to tell.

I reached the press site, and soon we had a report ready. We broke the story and two days later Shuttle Director Rich-ard Truly announced Challenger's crew cabin had been dis-covered, as we reported, about eighteen miles northeast of Cape Canaveral.

The following day, the USS Preserver put to sea and Navy divers began the grim task of recovering Challenger's crew cabin and the remains of the astronauts.

The crew compartment had hit the water with such force that, like a speeding bullet, it drilled a hole from the surface to the ocean's bottom, crushing itself nose down into the Atlantic's floor.

The bulkhead that kept the cabin air tight between the cargo bay and crew vessel faced the divers. Their first job was to remove it so they could reach the crew's remains.

The remains of Astronaut Judy Resnik were brought up first, followed by other remains from the flight deck. Then, from the mid deck, the remains of Teacher-In-Space Christa McAuliffe were brought to the surface, but others would have to wait for sections of the wreckage to be hauled onto the recovery ship.

On the decks of the USS Preserver its crew watched somberly as the twisted metal and dangling wires were pulled from beneath the water, hoisted onto the ship. It was a day to make sure every action was taken with respect for the remains of the seven heros.

All seemed to go well until the ship's steel cables tugged at a section of Challenger's mid deck. It appeared at first to be too much of a load. But, when it broke the surface, divers in the water and others on the deck froze. Suddenly a body in a blue astronaut jump suit floated on the surface of the sea, then it disappeared beneath the waves.

Minutes seemed to pass before the stunned recovery crew realized what had happened. They had lost Astronaut Gregory Jarvis, and some of the divers began a frantic search—a search that would not end for five weeks.

That night the USS Preserver slipped into Port Canaveral without running lights where two Air Force ambulances waited.

Across the port our NBC crew shot the somber scene, and when the ambulances pulled away from the dock, our crew, along with other cameramen and photographers, followed the medical vehicles through the towns of Cape Canaveral and Cocoa Beach to nearby Patrick Air Force Base.

When the ambulances parked at the base hospital, photographers were treated to a shocking surprise. The drivers opened their empty vehicles doors and told the news clan they were going home to bed.

The news people stared at each other. What happened to the astronauts' remains? Distrusting astronauts Bob Overmyer and Jim Bagian had managed a clandestine maneuver of their own. The part of the Challenger crew's remains that had been recovered had been loaded onto another vehicle and driven by secret route to the Patrick Air Force Base hospital.

The following morning, I reported on SUNRISE and the TODAY SHOW, the recovered remains were in the hospital.

NASA remained mute. Veteran astronauts Robert Crippen and Bob Overmyer felt strongly the news media could not be trusted and, in total secrecy, went about their assignment of supervising the recovery of the Challenger Seven.

To honor the fallen, a plan was presented where the other remains would be brought into port in flag-covered coffins with the ship's company in dress blues and standing at attention. But Robert Crippen would not permit it. He took secrecy to the extreme and ordered the unbelieving Captain of the USS Preserver *not* to execute the plan.

Robert Crippen's mistrust of the press made my job more difficult but not impossible.

As the recovery of the crew's remains moved ahead, and the search for Astronaut Gregory Jarvis' body continued without success, a new wrinkle was added to the recovery operation. The local Medical Examiner's office was making noises about how, under Florida law, it was that office's responsibility to determine cause of death within the state.

The local Medical Examiner was correct. That office could not vacate its responsibility for even the Challenger Seven. What if there were other deaths on federal property within NASA? What if there was a death due to an accident within a secret program? Could NASA, or the Air Force, be permitted to "cover up" these deaths? Investigate them on their own? Write one set of laws for themselves while everyone else had to obey the well-thought-out laws which have governed society for years?

I smelled a story. Jim Dick, the news producer of the

TODAY SHOW agreed. We aired the story the next morning and suddenly, Astronauts Robert Crippen and Bob Overmyer had a new problem.

The local press picked up the story, and my friend Hugh Harris had a "hot potato" in his hands for his Public Affairs' office.

Hugh, who I admire for his ability to remain cool under pressure and to quietly deal with things until a rational solution can be reached, made it known NASA had invited the local medical examiner to participate with the armed forces medical examiners who really had the "battle field" expertise necessary to identify the astronauts' remains.

The flap made Air Force officials at Patrick Air Force Base nervous, and they wanted the astronauts' remains out of their hospital.

"I don't want the autopsies performed on this base," Patrick Air Force Base Commander Nate Lindsey told NASA. "I want the job done on the Cape, where we have more security."

NASA officials agreed to remove the remains, but they knew if the word got out, the local Medical Examiner's office could intercept the remains and take possession.

"You'll just have to work around that," the base commander said.

"No sweat," Astronaut Joe Kerwin assured him. "We'll get the job done."

Brevard County Sheriff Jake Miller didn't really want anything to do with it, but his deputies were standing by to follow the orders of the Medical Examiner's office if called.

I learned local law enforcement wouldn't be needed. Astronauts' remains would not touch state soil.

For a moment his heart stopped. Dead ahead of them, swooping upward, a line of pelicans were playing follow-the-leader in a twilight sky. Their closing speed made the birds expand explosively in their view and then they were gone, rushing beneath the helicopter lifted upward instinctively by the pilot.

"Wow!" the copilot grinned as the helicopter settled down again, holding its true course for the Cape Canaveral Air Force station. "No heartstoppers, please. An accident we don't need."

"Not on this flight," the pilot grimly agreed, nodding his helmet toward the landscape below. "We wouldn't want the local smokies taking a look inside this plane."

Below them was the smooth, wide sandy coastline that is Cocoa Beach, and behind them was Patrick Air Force Base, but more importantly, with them, inside the helicopter, were the first recovered remains of the Challenger Seven.

The helicopter swept over Port Canaveral and out the window of the descending aircraft the crew could see the lights illuminating the row of tall rocket gantries growing larger with every passing second. In the distance, an important ship was approaching the port.

The pilot flared out in a gentle surge of power, and the plane made a feathery touchdown. The remains of Judy Resnik and Christa McAuliffe and some others were soon removed and on their way to the Life Sciences' hangar.

During the early evening of March 12th, 1986 the USS Preserver eased into Port Canaveral, running lights fully lit, carrying flag-covered coffins with part of its crew standing as an honor guard in full-dress-blues. Other crew members lined the deck at parade rest, all showing respect for more of the Challenger Seven's remains reclaimed from the sea.

A defiant Captain decided he, and only he, was commander of his vessel. He and his crew felt strongly that stone-headed secrecy was far down the list of importance. To them, as it was to the overwhelming majority of Americans, *respect* for the fallen headed the list.

Hundreds of local citizens, many workers at the space center, filled Jetty Park on the south side of the channel. Picnics were stopped, games ceased, Americans stood tall and applauded. Each were suddenly aware of what they were seeing. They were the taxpayers, the people, the owners of the shuttle fleet, the ones who pay for every nut and bolt NASA buys. The Challenger Seven rode into space, as do all astronauts, on their space ships, at their pleasure. Secrecy has its place. This wasn't it.

The applause was followed by quiet respect, and everyone quietly watched as the USS Preserver moved to a silent stop across the channel where seven Air Force ambulances waited.

I was never prouder.

In the coming days, while the search continued for Astronaut Greg Jarvis' body, armed forces pathologists identified the remains of six of the seven Challenger crew members.

Astronaut Robert Crippen was determined that when the remains were turned over to the families, there would be seven coffins, not six, and at one point, in an act of desperation, he hired a local scallop boat to drag its nets across the bottom of the ocean in hopes of finding the missing crew member.

On April 15th, when most hope had been abandoned, divers were busy collecting Challenger wreckage from the ocean's floor. About two hundred yards from where the crew cabin had been found, they stumbled onto Astronaut Jarvis' remains.

The seventh crew member was brought to the surface and his remains were placed with those of his mates.

The Challenger Seven had been reunited.

The initial and futile mission to find surviving astronauts evolved into a $100 million, seven-month effort to search the Atlantic for Challenger debris.

Air Force Colonel Edward O'Connor, who headed the recovery operation, said approximately 91,000 miles of the ocean's surface from Cape Canaveral to North Carolina, and 420 miles of its bottom, was searched in the great salvage effort.

For me, the recovery operation ended after seven months of high-stress, flat-out competition. It ended with me satisfied I had done my best. But my body felt like it had aged seven years instead of seven months and I still needed to train for the Journalist-in-Space Contest. Jogging seemed to be the answer, and with my home on the ocean, the sands of Cocoa Beach offered the perfect place to run.

ELEVEN

"Sudden Death"

A jogger doesn't begin his run with the thought that it will end in death. I surely didn't on May 28th, 1987. Those of us on the white sands of Cocoa Beach, Florida were enjoying a typical late spring day. The temperature was in the mid-eighties, and you could feel the first wave of approaching summer. Taut sails pushed riders on fast-moving wheels along the beach, while across the brilliant blue sea a cruise ship hung like a slow-moving cloud where the ocean and sky come together.

It was good to be home. As an NBC News Correspondent, I had just returned from covering the Challenger disaster, its aftermath and its recovery.

The grief of the weeping families of those killed was still fresh in my mind. I had never learned how to escape into the detached world of a reporter. Home, my regular routine, would help those memories fade.

I took a deep breath of salty air and, with long strides, crossed the walkover above the sand dunes that connect our backyard with the beach.

For ten years I had been a jogger. Now, it was even more important than ever. I had been selected as one of the eight southeastern finalists in the Journalist-in-Space project. There had been 1,705 applications from journalists which had now been whittled down to the final forty, and I knew that if I were to fly in space, I must keep in shape.

I felt my feet sink into the sand, and I stopped to push my body through a few stretching exercises—to get it limber for the run.

Three minutes passed and I was ready. I turned northward, into the wind, my steps increasing in stride as I walked briskly. A smile crossed my face as I felt the warm ocean breeze, smelled the clean, unpolluted sea air. Life was good.

Ten minutes later my body was ready. It was time to turn around, to face the south, to begin the run downwind. My legs moved in rhythm with the calls of the sea gulls that flew overhead.

Inside his chest, Jay Barbree's heart began to react to the increased demand for more blood. It pumped the oxygen-rich liquid to his leg and arm muscles, to his lungs, to his heart itself.

I could feel my body settling comfortably into the run. There was no stress, no extra effort. It was something I had done many times before, and it felt as natural as a late-evening stroll.

I let my mind drift into thoughts of the future, of sitting in the crew cabin of a Space Shuttle on its launch pad, waiting for blastoff with a frozen heartbeat, and how the heat of the Shuttle's ignition would thaw that frozen heartbeat, and how I would do my best to tell a worldwide radio and television audience what it was like to ride a pillar of fire through the gravity rapids to orbit.

I fantasized that my commentary would have an absolute candor of emotion, of sensation, fear, exuberance, wonder. How awesome it would be riding an express train of fire as the shuttle peeled away the layers of gravity. How my commentary would attempt to take the public along for the thundering ride through the sky, asking listeners to hold my hand as together we would tumble into weightlessness—asking them to stay with me for the thrill of swift sunrises and sunsets in orbit, and for the wonder of God's paintbrush as the awesome sights unfold before my eyes.

Within Barbree's body, a complex sequence of events was underway. As his feet pushed him across the sand, the muscles in his legs and arms continued to work harder. His lungs gulped more air. His heart beat faster. All demanded more oxygen-rich blood to meet increased energy demands and to remove by-products of the muscular activity.

Jogging for me was a time to think, to reflect on life, to give thanks.

I thought about how I had witnessed the Challenger blowup, how I had watched seven astronauts die in a sky filled with fire, steam, and jagged metal.

I was thankful for a healthy family.

I was thankful to be alive.

My feet continued to dig into the sand as I moved along the familiar beach. Home after home slipped past my view. I had seen them hundreds of times, knew most who lived in the salt-weathered structures.

Inside a body covered with sweat, Barbree's blood moved through the lungs to enrich itself with oxygen, and then into the left side of his heart, the muscle's major pumping chamber.

His heart rate was now in the 140s and the organ had increased its stroke volume to distribute blood to meet the growing needs of the body.

I ran past the Baptist Church, saying a quiet prayer as the familiar steeple crossed my view. The preselected turnaround point was just ahead.

I made the turnaround and began the trip back. My feet gripped the sand more firmly as my legs began their push into the wind. I could sense the change in my body, the demand for more energy.

As the heart continued to attempt to satisfy the body's demand, blood was now being kept away from those parts of the body not involved in the exercise.

The blood flow was being sent to the muscles being used,

*and additional blood flow was increased to the brain, skin,
and to the heart muscle itself.*

I was vaguely aware of the increasing strain on my
body, of the new energy demands. But there was no cause
for alarm. I felt the strain was due to the extra three pounds I
had gained.

*The workload on the heart continued to increase. Com-
pared to the demand for blood to the muscles involved in
sustaining his jogging, the flow of blood to sustain his heart
was sluggish and was controlled by only the small coronary
arteries.*

*The plaque obstructing the normal blood flow through
the coronaries was setting up a dangerous situation. Barbree's
oxygen-starved heart was functioning poorly as a pump.*

I could feel the heavier air, the humidity. I breathed
more rapidly, pulled more air into my burning lungs.

*The heart was doing its best to keep up with the body's
demands, with its own needs to be met.*

Ahead I could see the finish point. I was tired. More
tired than usual, but I was determined to finish my run.

*What Barbree didn't know was that the heart was now
beating at a rate of 160 strokes per minute, trying to keep the
body supplied with its demand for blood, trying to draw
enough flow through its own plaque-clogged coronary arteries
to supply its own needs.*

I checked my watch. The run was twenty-five minutes
old. Just ahead, just past home, was the finish point.

*Inside the chest his blood-starved heart became irritable.
Its electrical field was disturbed. An electrical seizure caused
the heart to beat irregularly.*

I crossed the finish line twenty-seven minutes after my run began. Tired, very tired. But pleased. I had finished. It was time to begin the walk down.

The chaotically beating heart could not reorganize. It desperately needed more blood. Its clogged arteries could not handle its additional requirements. Death was only seconds away.

I was not aware of what was going on inside my chest. There was no pain. Only exhaustion.

I looked up at our house, at the gray walkover above the sand dunes leading to the backyard. Suddenly, there was a flutter inside. I could feel my heart jerking, refusing to beat with a smooth rhythm. Instantly I knew something was wrong. There had been no warning.

Inside, the heart was entering ventricular fibrillation. The electrical seizure was causing it to beat in a rapid, unsynchronized, uncoordinated fashion. It was no longer pumping blood. It seemed like a bundle of squirming worms.

My knees felt weak. My body went limp. I fell on my side with my arm resting under my head. Suddenly there was only blackness. A pure, deep blackness, absent of dreams.

The heart quivered to a stop. It refused to beat. Doctors call it "sudden death."
Jay Barbree knew nothing. He was dead.

TWELVE

"The Revival"

*T*he little girl stared at the stilled body of the man collapsed on the sand. She snickered as she watched the surf wash foam around his jogging shoes.

"Look at the funny man, Mommy," she snickered again. "He's getting his shoes all wet."

The woman ran up to the child. "C'mon, baby," she said, grasping the little girl's arm and leading her away. "He's drunk, honey," she scolded. "Stay away from him."

Others near Jay Barbree's lifeless body paid little notice. It wasn't all that unusual to see a person lying on the sand, but it was unusual to see a man drop before their eyes. Puzzling, but not alarming to most who made it a practice not to get involved.

About a block south, David Frank, an engineer for RCA, was well into his daily walk. He was headed north, approaching the lifeless form.

"My God," he spoke to no one. "That guy just jogged by me."

He hurried and knelt beside Barbree, saw eyes staring into space. He felt for a pulse. There was none.

Frank had spent many years on the Eastern Missile Range, assigned to tracking stations where CPR was learned by most. Where doctors and trained medical personnel were a scarcity. He knew what had to be done.

149

Quickly he began CPR. Pumping the chest and blowing air into the lungs.

A minute passed. He stopped. Barbree coughed, tried to breathe on his own. No luck. The breathing stopped again.

David Frank turned, looking for help. "Call the Rescue Squad," he signaled a passerby.

*O*ne block north Pat Sullivan, a college student, was at work at the restaurant "Coconuts." He was carrying supplies into the dining room when he noticed the small group of people standing around Barbree's body.

"What's going on down there?" he yelled to a man on the beach.

"It looks like a drowning to me," the man replied.

Sullivan turned to his fellow workers. "Any of you know CPR?"

None responded.

"Here, take this," he said, handing a case of beer to a coworker. "I know CPR. I'll go."

The slim, young man went down the steps two at a time, and ran the block to where David Frank was standing.

He stared at the lifeless body on the beach and, gasping for air, he froze. "My God," he shouted. "It's Mr. Barbree."

"You know him?" David Frank asked.

"I sure do," the young man responded. "His daughter, Karla, and I have been friends ever since we were freshmen in High School." He turned, pointing. "They live right up there, that house on the ocean."

He turned back. Stared at Barbree's face, a purple face absent of life.

"He's dead. I just know he's dead," he whispered to himself.

He looked at David Frank. "Let's do what we can," he told the older man. "You give him mouth-to-mouth, and I'll handle the compressions."

The two men started to work. They managed to prevent damage to the brain and vital organs by manually pumping blood through the body.

*T*he attempted rivival of Jay Barbree was taking place within
the shadows of the Park Place Condominium.

   In a unit on the third floor, Debi Hall was busy preparing
dinner, annoyed with her detective husband for leaving the
police radio on. The constant 10-4s and law enforcement
chatter were getting on her nerves.

   She paid scant attention to the call that a man was down
on the beach and the Rescue Squad was rolling, until she
heard the location.

   Then, she ran to the balcony, looked down and saw two
men working on a lifeless body.

   On her way out the door, she only stopped long enough
to turn off the stove.

   Her reaction was a normal one for Debi. She had been
trained as an emergency medical technician to quickly react
to any life-threatening situation. Her job was to take care of
workers on the nation's spaceport at the Kennedy Space Center, including the astronauts.

   Within seconds she was on the beach, moving Pat Sullivan and David Frank aside.

   First, she checked for a pulse. There was none. Then she
resumed CPR. She knew it was critical to keep oxygen and
blood moving to the brain and other vital organs.

   She completed a sequence and shouted in Barbree's ear.
"Don't go to the light! Don't go to the light! You're gonna' be all
right."

   Her efforts were tireless. She kept the rhythm going.
"Where the hell is that Rescue Squad?" she yelled.

*E*d Clemons and Lee Proctor were busy with firehouse
maintenance duties when the call came in. They both
stopped, and looked at each other. Clemons, a paramedic,
had seen it all too often before, and the outcome was all too
predictable. But they had to do what they could. Once in a
great while they did get lucky, and maybe this call would be
that rare lucky one.

   One thing in the victim's favor, he was lucky enough to

drop within a block of the Cocoa Beach Fire Station and the city's Rescue Squad.

Proctor took the wheel and the rescue unit screamed out of the fire house and headed for the beach. There was only one traffic light, and the emergency switcher took care of it. They raced onto the beach, came to a complete stop, their eyes searching.

The only activity was to the south, and they burned sand to the location, where Clemons was immediately on the ground by the lifeless body.

He stared at a man dressed in jogging shoes, dry shorts and a shirt wet with sweat.

"This guy didn't drown," he protested to his partner. "He's a jogger."

"That's right," Debi Hall told them. "He went into v-fib while jogging."

Her eyes darted back and forth between the two firemen. "Did you bring a defib pack?"

"No," Clemons said. "The ambulance is on its way with that gear."

He read the disgust in Debi Hall's face, but let it pass as he prepared to go to work.

He and Proctor took over, first checking for a pulse. It still wasn't there.

Clemons reached for an airway tube, moved Barbree's tongue out of the way.

"He's got chewing gum in his mouth," Debi told the paramedic, as she leaned her head near the stricken man.

"Don't go to the light," she screamed in Barbree's ear. "Stay here with us. You're gonna' be all right. Don't go to the light."

"What's wrong with this woman?" Clemons mumbled. "She's in my way."

The paramedic turned, signaled to police sergeant Duane Hinkley to clear the area. They did not know Debi Hall was a certified emergency medical technician from the space center.

Clemons instructed his partner, Lee Proctor, to begin CPR chest compressions again while he removed the gum and inserted the airway tube.

Next he attached a blue ambu-bag with an oxygen bottle

to the tube, and for the first time since Barbree collapsed, the man's lungs were being enriched with oxygen.

Lee Proctor continued his steady rhythm of chest compressions which were manually moving the blood through the stilled heart into the lungs to pick up the fresh oxygen and send it to the brain and other organs.

Barbree's color began to return and occasionally he would attempt to breathe, what medical people call agonal respiration.

The rescue work continued until the ambulance arrived with the defibrillators.

Emergency medical technician Chris Bedard leaped from the vehicle with the defibrillator pack and immediately checked for a pulse. Still there was none.

He reached for the eyelids and checked the pupils. Good, he thought. They haven't dilated.

Bedard and his partner hooked leads to Barbree's chest and checked the monitor. The screen displayed what appeared to be chicken scratchings, but it told the medical team Barbree's heart was in ventricular fibrillation, disorganized electrical patterns causing the organ to quiver instead of pumping normally.

"Stand back," Bedard ordered as Barbree's shirt was removed and the defibrillator's paddles were placed on his chest.

Bedard set the equipment for 200 joules shock, and the 200 newtons of electrical energy lifted the stricken man's body several inches above the sand.

The jolt did nothing. The monitor continued to display the pattern indicating ventricular fibrillation.

Bedard set the equipment for a heavier force—300 joules shock. Again the electrical energy jolted Barbree's body off the ground.

Nothing.

The equipment was reset for a third shock, more energy, 360 joules.

Again Barbree's body was jolted into suspension above the sand.

Still nothing.

*Bedard looked at the others. "Continue CPR," he ordered,
moving to get an IV needle in one of Barbree's arms.*

*He started heart stimulant drugs into the blood stream as
fresh oxygen continued to flow into the lungs. The CPR moved
the drugs and fresh blood into the heart muscle itself.*

*While the medics worked feverishly to revive Jay Barbree,
life in his home only one hundred yards away continued unaware that he had fallen victim to sudden death.*

*The Barbree family had only moved into the seaside
house four months before, and his wife, Jo, was still busy
decorating. She was painting a household item in the garage
when she first heard a noise, the sound of someone banging
on the back windows.*

*She stopped painting. Listened. The banging moved to
the side windows, and as she stepped from the garage, she
saw Pat Sullivan standing there, face white.*

*"Mrs. Barbree, your husband has fallen on the beach," he
blurted the words.*

*"Whaaattt???" she screamed as she began running along
the house toward the ocean.*

*The young man ran after her, grabbing her arm. "Don't
run," he ordered. "The professionals are there. They are taking care of him," he added, slowing her to a walk. "We don't
need you to fall down and hurt yourself too."*

*Jo's mind was now numb. She paid little attention to
what Pat was saying. All she could think about was that Jay
had had a heart attack, just like his brother Larry, just like all
of his family. The Barbree curse, she thought.*

*She reached the backyard and started over the dunes
overpass; to her left she could see the small crowd, the Fire
Department's rescue vehicle next to the county ambulance.*

*She picked up her pace, almost running again, but when
she and the young man reached the scene she could see little
for the crowd.*

*Pat Sullivan kept her back until she heard Chris Bedard
say, "Let's get him in the ambulance. We've done all we can
for him here."*

She watched as her husband was loaded into the vehicle, and she felt someone's hand on her shoulder. "I'll take you to the hospital, Mrs. Barbree," Sergeant Duane Hinkley said.

She looked at the large police officer. "Thank you," she attempted a smile, "but first I have to lock the house."

The medics continued the procedures inside the ambulance to keep Barbree's brain and other organs enriched with fresh blood as the vehicle, sirens screaming, raced from the beach and down A1A toward the hospital.

Ed Clemons sat in the front, still assisting Chris Bedard who continued to search his mind for his next move. "Let's hit him with the paddles again," he said.

Bedard kept the defibrillator set at 360 joules, and with everyone clear, he sent another shock of electrical energy through Barbree's chest.

They stared at the monitor. A heartbeat. Not perfect, but a heartbeat.

The unorganized electrical field in the heart had responded. It had been reorganized by the electrical shock and, although not perfect, the heart was pumping again. There was a pulse, and a blood pressure was returning.

The medics stared at each other. Their lips stretched into economy-size grins. "I don't know who you are, buddy," Chris Bedard laughed, "but you are one lucky sucker."

"Welcome back from the dead," another said quietly.

Ed Clemons spoke up. "This is one time we won, guys." He shook his head. "Not often, but this once."

"We're not outta' the woods yet," Bedard reminded them.

"Nope, but it's a hell of a start," Clemons grinned.

They sat quietly for the rest of the ride, tracing the restored heartbeat across the monitor. Each knew if it had not been for the CPR efforts of David Frank, Pat Sullivan, and Debi Hall before their arrival, there was no way they would have won this day.

The facts are that only twenty-five to thirty percent of "sudden deaths" are brought back with the immediate attention of trained emergency medical technicians. But by the time they reached the Cape Canaveral Hospital, Barbree was fighting back.

He was taken to the emergency room where his survival instincts made him combative. He fought nurses' and doctors' efforts to restrain him, to keep tubes down his throat, needles in his arm.

A worried wife waited anxiously outside. What was she going to do if he died. Their youngest was in college, and even though Jay had provided for his family, there were many decisions still to be made, if this was an abrupt end to the life they had lived together for twenty-six years.

She turned to Sergeant Hinkley. "You think he's dead?" she asked flatly.

The veteran police officer, who would within months be brought down by a suspect's bullet and have his own battle to hold onto life, somberly looked into her worried face. "I'll see what's going on," he said.

Sergeant Hinkley moved to the door of the emergency room, looked in, and a smile crossed his face.

He turned back, walked to where Jo Barbree was sitting. "Hell no, he's not dead," he grinned. "He's in there giving them hell right now. They're having trouble holding him down."

Inside the room Jay Barbree twisted and turned, trying to make sense of his predicament.

Where did all the fog come from?

That's not fog, you idiot!

The hell it isn't! It's too cold not to be fog.

No, wait, let me think about it. Think? How can I think with all that noise. Why don't those people shut up?

There. That's it. It's moving away.

Shut up you people!

Why can't I hear my words? Hell, I don't know. Yes I do. There's something in my throat.

Look at the stars. My God, they are bright. The blackness. What a blackness. I've never seen night like this before. Never stars so bright.

He turned toward the light.

But it's not night over there. Over there it is beautiful. If I could go over there I could get away from this noise.

He struggled for a moment, then lay back exhausted.

I'm too tired to go now. I'll rest for awhile. Rest in the blackness.

I fell back into the dark pit, back into the sleep without dreams, only to be awakened again by the noise, by a radio playing gut bucket rock, and by those loud people.

It seemed so out of place, all the noise among the bright stars, within the peaceful blackness.

I turned to the beauty. The grass reached out, beckoning to me. The earth itself was alive and it flowed to me, and the trees were living creatures, green-golden-silver, swaying into a canopy through which there shone a glorious golden light.

Was this death?

Was this my death?

Was I moving closer to . . .

To what? To my family my death would be a shock. To me it would be the loss of my darling wife, the loss of my daughters, of my son, of my grandchildren—the loss of dying gently in my own bed at age eighty, surrounded by those you love. To my friends my death would bring the titillation of regret along with relief that it had not been them. To my colleagues it would be a few lines of newspaper space, a brief mention on an hourly newscast, possibly a line or two read by Tom Brokaw on Nightly News, a passing mention on TODAY about my years of service to NBC News. To anyone else . . . Good Lord, there wasn't anyone else.

So what? No passion, no anger. It was all too much, too quickly. My body shuddered. No pain.

I could *feel* life draining from me, but it was being replaced, and the thought whispered through my mind that nothing in life, nothing between heaven and earth, is really lost, and there was comfort in that when the light appeared as a tiny speck in the darkness, a light swelling in size and in brilliance, filling an endless globe of darkness, yet translucent and becoming a cross to fill the world and the universe beyond. A universe which stretched before me forever. It shone from within, and I thought of God.

I was alone.

Drifting in space.

Alone?

But suddenly out of the light, out of its magnificent brilliance there appeared a darker form, a bed, a huge bed being pushed by two white shadowed forms, two nurses, and I heard the gallop of their feet, the high-pitched squeal of unoiled wheels . . .

The brilliant light vanished.

It was gone.

There was only the huge bed, the nurses taking tremendous strides, crashing through the darkness, the squealing wheels screaming in my brain.

An invisible hand grasped me, swept me like a leaf in a high wind, hurled me after the fleeing nurses.

Instantly the bed and the nurses stopped, and I suddenly realized there was someone in the bed. A man. A familiar man, and he turned his head to face me.

Me. It was me. I was in the bed, but I wasn't. How could this be?

Where are we going? I asked in my silent voice.

"We're going to CIC."

What's that? Another voice asked?

"Cardiac Intensive Care."

I moved into the huge bed, into my body, into a body strapped to the railings with arms loaded with I.V.s, with a mouth filled with tubes.

Suddenly we were moving again, but not across the universe. We were moving down a long hall, moving by people, by equipment, and in step with disassociated sounds.

Sleep—I drifted into it. It was time for the tranquility and peace.

T HIRTEEN

"A Second Life"

Now the light was distant, not in focus. It faded and returned with much difficulty. It refused to remain in place, or to stay for more than a slow moment. I tried to go to it, but I couldn't move. Suddenly, I realized why! Hydra! The monstrous serpent with nine heads was wrapped around my arms, my legs, around my body, and her obedient snakes squirmed in my throat, wiggled out of my mouth.

I fought to free myself, tried desperately to cough the snakes from my throat. Nothing worked. I was chained to a single spot in the universe.

I tried to relax. Think, Jay, I scolded myself. Focus on the distant light. Force it to move, to come closer. Bring it to you. But I couldn't.

Suddenly there were voices, unrecognizable voices mixed with other strange sounds. They grew in volume and I heard one that was familiar. The voice of my wife, Jo, of my partner, of my best friend, of my only "bunkie."

I tried to go to the voice, tried to reach her, but Hydra wouldn't let go. The monster's nine serpentine bodies held firm.

"Don't fight it, Jay," she spoke softly, her voice distant, her words separated in time. "Your arms and legs are tied down, the doctors have tubes down your throat. Don't try to talk."

My eyes blinked open and I stared at her, eyes wide, my

159

muscles challenging Hydra's grip. But, wait! It wasn't Hydra restraining me now. It was nurses.

I relaxed.

"You fell unconscious on the beach," my wife said. "Everything is all right now. The doctors are taking care of you. It's all right, honey . . . It's all right . . ."

Her words trailed away as I slept again.

A short time later I heard Jo speaking and I moved through the darkness toward her voice.

"Don't let the machines scare you, Jay," she said softly.

Scare me? Why would they scare me?

"It's the monitors," she said quietly, her hand stroking my hair which was still full of sand.

I felt safe—confused, but safe, and with each passing moment the sounds became clearer. I could hear the repetitious beep, beep, beep, but suddenly I realized I wasn't in my bed. It was someone else's bed. A strange, white bed, rock hard.

Not to worry. Jo was there. My beautiful beauty queen, the mother of my children, my life-long partner. I floated back to sleep.

I spent the first two days in the hospital my body inhabited by tubes, fighting restraints, trying to remember. I kept waking up and writing on a pad one question: What happened?

My wife would tell me and I would promptly forget.

My brain was literally swollen. The minutes it had been deprived of oxygen-rich-blood had caused it to swell and the doctors said I wouldn't be fully conscious until the swelling went down.

The question was how long would it take me to remember, and would I ever really recall any of the events surrounding my "sudden death."

The answer was yes; I was recalling them, but slowly. There was the confusion between the real and the unreal dreams. But after two days I was far enough back so that they removed the restraints, removed the tubes from my throat. It left me more alert and hungry.

The first food I was permitted was some leftover cold chicken wings and cheeses from an afternoon hospital party.

The food was stale and greasy, but I was so hungry it was a king's feast to me. And when I had finished, my wife brought in the local newspaper from the day before.

I opened it to page one and read the headline:

VETERAN SPACE REPORTER STRICKEN WHILE JOGGING

My eyes moved to the first paragraph:

> NBC correspondent and space launch veteran Jay Barbree, 53, suffered an apparent heart attack Thursday while jogging near his home in Cocoa Beach.

"I did not," I protested to my wife. "I haven't had a heart attack. I passed out, that's all."

"Well, they're not sure, yet," Jo said, trying to soothe me. "The doctors are still waiting for some test results."

"Well, I'm sure," I said. "I feel as strong now as ever, and there's no pain. None."

I turned my attention back to the story,"

> Barbree, who has covered the space program for 29 years and is the only journalist to have witnessed every manned and unmanned launch, was listed in serious but stable condition in the intensive care unit at . . .

I stopped reading. For the first time my situation was taking on a more serious meaning to me. Could I have had a heart attack? Could all of the prevention, all of the measures I had taken over the years to avoid one, gone for naught?

No, they hadn't. This I was sure of in my own mind, and when the doctors returned, they returned with good news. All the tests were in and there was no sign of heart damage. I had fallen into "sudden death" because of apparent ventricular fibrillation. The question was, what had triggered it?

The doctors decided further study was needed to find out why, and ordered me to continue resting, continue climbing out of my pit of lost memory.

I had lost only about a day and the doctors kept telling me how lucky I was, how no more than one in four are brought back, with the best of care, from "sudden death."

But I was, and I am still of the simple opinion that somebody up there likes me. For me, death was not frightening. It was, in fact, peaceful. Somehow I knew it wasn't time. I felt then, and still do, there is something left for me to do.

It may be something simple, or it could be an overwhelming task. Whatever, that someone up there who likes me, who watches over and takes care of us, will help me see that its done.

And about being lucky. I've always been lucky, really. Not lucky rich. A farm boy born *lucky* poor. A satisfying sort of luck. Luck that saw I was one of three out of two hundred fifty who made it into the Air Force, luck that put me in position to finish my education, luck that had me at Cape Canaveral at the right time to land the NBC News job, luck that helped me understand and file a winning application in the Journalist-in-Space project. Luck that saw that I drop dead near EMTs (Emergency Medical Technicians). Just pure and simple luck.

The longer I lay in the hospital bed strapped to the heart monitors, the clearer my thoughts grew. I was coming to realize that if I was going to survive, to stay clear of another episode of "sudden death," then I must get control of my emotions, restrain my hostility. I must understand that the world is inhabited by a variety of people, assholes as well as saints, and long after I depart this earth, the planet will still have its share of both.

I laughed as I reminded myself that some people would think there was one less asshole here when I left.

My wife, Jo, lifted her eyes from the magazine she was reading and asked, "What are you laughing about?"

"Oh, nothing," I grinned.

"You must be feeling good," she said, moving from her chair to sit on the side of my hospital bed.

"I feel fine," I assured her. "I haven't been in pain."

"You're not sore where they shocked you with the paddles?"

"Nope, not a bit," I answered, running my fingers across my chest.

Jo smiled and moved back to her chair in the corner, and I returned to my thoughts, to reappraisal of myself.

The fact that I had not felt pain was somewhat of a mystery, and I couldn't let go of the nagging question of why there wasn't a warning? I had always assumed that if I ever overdid it jogging, then my body would warn me, my heart would transmit a pain telling me to slow down, to take it easy. But it didn't. There had been no pain, no warning.

This was a fact of which all joggers should be aware; a fact for anyone who exercises strenuously.

"Pistol Pete" Maravich, Astronauts Donn Eisele and Jim Irwin, jogging guru Jim Fixx, and many others also had no warning. They too had been stricken while jogging.

If anyone had cautioned me before I fell on the beach, I would have paid them little mind. I was convinced I was invincible and I was equally convinced I must do battle over every little disagreement. You wouldn't catch Jay Barbree walking around a fight.

That conviction, I knew, was not only an inherited trait, but was also a product of my roots. Farm people, for the most part, are independent and proud, ready to settle their own disagreements. No arbitrator need apply, no judge is needed.

Long before I jogged on the beach, I would jog along the bicycle path that lined the main street to our home, with dogs nipping at my feet. There's just something about the bare legs of a jogger that seems to trigger canines, and those

who were permitted to roam free in spite of the city's leash
law were a problem.

There was one dog in particular that went crazy each
time he saw me.

One Sunday morning, the streets of Cocoa Beach were
quiet, and I was well into my run when I reached the house
where the dog lived. His owner was outside mowing the
lawn and the gate to the backyard had been left opened. No
sooner than I reached the corner of the property, the dog
came charging out of the back yard, clamping down on my
right ankle with a full bite.

His owner paid no notice as I shouted at the dog, hitting
at him, trying to make him turn my ankle loose. I screamed
at the owner to call his dog off, but the man just kept mowing his grass, ignoring his dog's attack on me.

The dog broke the skin and blood was running down
my leg. The pain was becoming unbearable. With my bloody
right foot, I brought my best Karate kick, developed from
years of study in Aikido, full force to the dog's stomach. The
foot lifted the animal off the ground, sending him sailing
back into his yard.

"Hey, you sonfabitch," the man screamed, stopping his
mower. "You kicked my dog."

"You bastard," I screamed back. "This isn't the first time
your dog bit me. Why didn't you call him off?"

"You sissy ass joggers should be bit," he said, walking
toward me in a threatening manner.

"Keep coming, asshole," I shouted. "Come on over here
on public property and I'll show you what a sissy I am."

My temper was now at "boil over," and I was ready to
plant this asshole in his lawn. What he didn't know was that
I had spent seven years achieving the rank of Shodan (first
degree black belt in the martial art of Aikido), and I was
ready to put that training to use. I had had to use it a couple
of times in covering civil rights issues, but this was different.
I was in a mood to kill this uncaring sonfabitch who obviously thought his dog had the right to feed off joggers.

The man suddenly stopped in his yard, appearing to
sense he was biting off more than he could chew.

"Come on," I screamed. "Come on, fat man, I want you."

He stayed planted in his tracks. "I'm calling the police," he said.

"Whatta' you gonna' tell 'em?" I yelled. "Your dog bit me? You gonna' tell 'em your dog's off his leash?"

"You didn't have a right to kick 'em," he said in a nervous tone.

"You stupid sonfabitch," I screamed. "I'm on public property. Your dog is not on a leash. If he bites me again, I'll stuff'im for you and you can mount him on your wall."

The dog had long since departed and found a hiding place in the back yard. His owner suddenly decided to join him. "Whatta' you running from a sissy jogger for?" I screamed after him. "Why don't you and your dog come back? I'm only a sissy. No reason to be afraid."

A few minutes later my temper began to cool, and I started to get control of myself. I knew I should call the police, let them handle it, but I was used to settling my own arguments. I wasn't in the least aware of the damage my anger was doing to my coronary heart disease, and I simply didn't care. I was fighting a battle of right over wrong, and what was important to me was that I win.

My bleeding ankle wouldn't permit me to run, so I began limping back toward the house, where Jo dressed it.

"You ought to go to the hospital," she murmured worriedly.

"No need for that," I said. "It'll heal."

"What about rabies?"

"No chance, not the way that dog is pampered."

After that, I began carrying a heavy stick with me each time I jogged on the streets, and I no longer had a problem with dogs. But I still had my problem with a quick temper, with hostile reactions, especially in traffic.

It seemed to me that every slow driver on earth would receive a signal that Barbree was on the road and would hurry to their cars to block my path. I got to the point where the family hated to ride with me, although generally, when my hostility had cooled, we found my battles on the highway more comical than serious.

There was one incident where even my famous temper was forced to back down. This tourist decided to stop in the middle of the road on A1A in downtown Cocoa Beach to check his map. I came out of my car, screaming louder than a New York City taxi cab driver, and when the tourist decided to get out of his car, he kept getting and getting and getting. When he was finally out, he stood a head taller than me, and I'm six-feet-two.

The kids started laughing and I found that the best course of action. I too laughed, saying, "Uh uh, you're too damn big."

Of course I'm not the only person with a quick temper. I remember a neighbor of ours when I was a child. His name was Charlie Murkerson, and he went through life with a short fuse.

One day Charlie came in from the fields at noon for the meal we called "dinner," and after he had watered the team and given the mules their feed, he entered the house to learn his dinner wasn't ready.

Charlie roared into one of his usual screaming tirades, reminding his wife, Gracie, how hard he worked to put food on the table for the family, and the least he should expect is that there would be some of that food on the table when he took his noon break.

Gracie wasn't impressed. She had heard it all too often before, and she ignored Charlie's screaming and continued getting his dinner ready for the table.

Charlie grabbed the 12-gauge-shotgun off the wall, stomped out of the kitchen, shouting, "It's no use. There's no respect for me in this house anymore."

He ran down the steps and across the yard. "I'll just kill myself," he screamed with even a louder pitch in his voice as he disappeared behind the smokehouse.

Still, Gracie wasn't buying his threat. She had also heard the "I'm gonna kill myself" routine before.

Suddenly there was quiet, but just for a moment before the peace was broken with "Barooooooom!"

Gracie screamed, "Oh, my God," at the sound of the shotgun blast.

She ran out the door toward the smokehouse only to see Charlie peek around the building. When he saw he had her concerned, he shouted, "Bring me another shell, Gracie, I missed myself."

I chuckled at my own story.

Jo glanced up from her magazine again, shook her head gently. "You *are* in a good mood today," she smiled. "It's good to see you laugh."

"It's good to get those tubes out of my throat," I answered, suddenly reminded again of my good luck by the vision before me.

I looked at her, watched as she rubbed her shoulder muscles, I knew her neck must ache from sitting in that uncomfortable hospital chair for the past three days. But I had not expected her to be anywhere else.

Some men spend their lives searching for a mate. Some are looking for love. Some are looking for devotion. Others are looking for a friend. Most are looking for beauty. Well, I smiled, I had found them all, in this wonderful lady.

My mother, who loved Jo as much as she did any of her daughters, used to tell me, "Usually beauty is only skin deep, son, but in Jo's case, it's all the way to the bone." Then she would grin and add, "And in your case, Son, ugly on you is just as deep."

I laughed again. I didn't really have to be reminded that July 4th, 1958 was one of my luckiest days.

I was working for the local station then and I had been assigned to cover the Miss Brevard County Beauty Contest. The event was a traditional Fourth celebration. There was plenty of food, bands, speeches, and a bevy of beauties dressed in bathing suits, moving gracefully before the table of judges, and when the contest was over, I found myself trying to pronounce the name Reisinger.

A raven-haired beauty had won and I was getting ready to report the outcome live on the local station. Her first name, Jo, was no problem.

"It's pronounced *rye*, like rye bread," another reporter told me, and I went on the air without the slightest hint I had just seen, and was reporting a story involving, my future wife.

The coming months would find me covering other beauty contests—Miss Space, Miss Orbit, Miss whatever— and Jo Reisinger kept winning, but not with just her looks and her figure. She was also winning with her personality, her desire to be helpful and fair to others. And when it came time for the senior class to graduate, Jo was elected Homecoming Queen.

We were married a year and three months later, and through the years she has been by my side, never demanding life go her way, content to follow the path I've chosen, never resenting my selfishness, giving us daughters Alicia and Karla, and giving us dear son, Scott who was with us only two days.

That was a time that brought Jo and me closer together for all these good years, years that were now threatened, years that were also a portrait of a stressed-out life.

I wondered. Could the stress have been the sole contributor to my brush with death?

No, I answered my own question. It was only part of it. Heredity was the major culprit. That much I knew. But what else, I had to know.

My eyes moved back to Jo. Lovingly, I studied her. It was clear if we were to continue our life, any life, then it was time to assess the damage, to understand what happened, to set out on a new road to correct the faults of the past.

Doctors Rajan, Scharff, and Messersmith arrived with smiles, pleased with the progress I was making, and pleased with a plan they had. The tests they had ordered performed during the past forty-eight hours showed no heart damage. It had not been a heart attack, but the major question was what brought on the sudden heart failure? Was it a problem within my heart's electrical field? Was it self-induced by overexertion during my run? Or was it some other unknown possibility?

The doctors told me they had concluded that the man who could answer the questions was Dr. Onkar Narula who practiced at Cedars Medical Center in Miami. They explained he was a Clinical Professor of Cardiology at the University of Miami Medical School, one of the world's leading authorities on coronary arrhythmias and the author of several text books on the subject.

"We have his text books in our office," Dr. Scharff smiled.

"We use them, too," Dr. Messersmith added.

Doctors Norbett Scharff and Donald Messersmith were first on my case when I was brought into the hospital, and their advice, along with Dr. Rajan's, was critical.

"We think Onkar Narula is the man to pinpoint your problem, Jay," Dr. Rajan assured me, squeezing my hand.

"When do we get out of Dodge?" I smiled.

"Pardon me?"

"When do we go?"

"Oh, tomorrow," Dr. Rajan nodded. "Cedars will have a bed for you tomorrow."

Jo took my hand. "Liz at the Miami Bureau has arranged for an air ambulance, Jay. They'll fly you down."

"Narula is the top gun, huh?"

"That's right," Dr. Rajan assured me again.

"Well," I laughed. "As I said, partners, come sunup, we're getting out of Dodge."

FOURTEEN

"What Happened?"

We fell toward the upthrusting cloud world born in mid-day over southern Florida. The first tremors of heat bumped against the Beach Baron and my hands moved of their own accord to tighten my seat belt. Stupid, I thought, glancing up at the nurse and doctor on board the air ambulance. They had secured me firmly to the stretcher before we took off. I smiled at them and turned my gaze once again to the small window. After four days in that hospital, two days spent tied to the bed with tubes down my throat, I was sore, uncomfortable, and impatient to be done with the bumpy flight, to plant my feet solidly on ground.

I smiled inwardly. Fat chance of that. They wouldn't even let me walk from the ambulance to the plane. Hell, I never felt stronger in my life, but they wouldn't hear of it, and I was sure they wouldn't change their minds when we reached Miami.

My thoughts turned to what lay ahead, to my health, to my prospects for a life. What life? What kind of life? Must I live as an invalid? Would I be able to return to work? What would be the smart thing to do? Retire? Try to live without worry? Would this guarantee me a future? I didn't have the answers.

I turned to the window as the Beach Baron banked steeply, turning toward the ocean, and I focused on what I could see below. South Florida's countryside . . . murky, heavily thatched with cypress, cabbage palms, reeds, with sawgrass verdant in the rain-rich spring, followed by reflections leaping along the surface where before I could not see water. Then Australian pines, standing fortress-like on each side of twin concrete ribbons running north and south. Florida's Turnpike slashing its way along the gold coast.

Suddenly my ears felt stuffed. I pinched my nose and popped them. We were descending toward Miami International and the passage through the air brought even more familiar sights. The Tamiami Trail cutting its way across the edge of the everglades, a speeding air boat parting the tall sawgrass, swamp reeds, and cattails, cane-pole-fishermen lining a narrow canal, walls of dikes operated by the water management folks, cattle in the distance. After nearly thirty-years in Florida, there was little I hadn't seen.

Then, a sudden flash of light and I blinked. Bright sun against the surface of the intercoastal waterway. Miami coming up.

The Beach Baron rolled out of its final turn with the runway now straight ahead. Streets, traffic, stucco dwellings came into view. A blurred outline of wings moving ghostlike over the ground. Touchdown only seconds away.

The wheels kissed the concrete lightly and made a smooth bounce back into the air before coming down heavily on the runway, slamming my body into the stretcher as the small twin aircraft was braked hard for a turn into a taxiway. Busy Miami International has little time to give to private planes, and the Beach Baron was soon at its ramp where I was unloaded into an ambulance and enroute to Cedars Medical Center.

We sped along streets, siren screaming. I turned to the attendant. "Hell, I'm not dying,' I said. "I did that four days ago."

He laughed. "If we don't run with the siren, we'll never get there in this traffic."

"I've often suspected you guys of doing this," I grinned.

"More than you know," he nodded, still smiling.

The driver drove the ambulance into a winding drive, stopping before a group of buildings, one with its floors stair-stepped pyramid style toward the sky. "This it?" I asked.

"Yep, Cedars Medical Center," the attendant answered.

I was mildly surprised to find the center "used." Not rundown, not decaying, but used. It was lacking in up-to-date fixtures, and when we went inside I saw it was "used" because it was a busy center, a private, not-for-profit international center to treat acute diseases.

So, this is where the "top gun" practices medicine, I thought as the attendants delivered me to my room.

I was mildly surprised to find an international hospital staff. Jamaican and Cuban nurses, Bahamian technicians, others from other Caribbean nations, even a few from South America and Europe.

There was also, of course, some local talent, and once I had settled in, I learned Cedars was affiliated with the University of Miami School of Medicine, and it was equipped to use the latest technological advances. In fact, six hundred fifty physicians practice in Cedars in a full range of medical and surgical specialties with an emphasis on neurosurgery, microsurgery, oncology, and most important to me, cardiology.

Only minutes had passed when a pleasant young lady with a Latin accent came into my room. She smiled. "Good morning, I'm Dr. Salis."

"Good morning, Doctor."

"How are we feeling?"

"Great," I answered. "A little sore from lying in these hard hospital beds, but I'm rested and feel just great."

"Any chest pains?"

"None," I answered, moving to sit up. "In fact, Doctor, I never had any."

She went on to explain she was Dr. Narula's assistant, and she was there to take down my medical history.

When she was done she asked, "Any questions?"

"I understand Dr. Narula is the best?" I smiled.

"Absolutely," she assured me. "I'm very lucky to work with him, to learn."

"What kind of record does he have in the catheterization lab?"

"What do you mean?"

"What is his percentage of loss?"

THE DAY I DIED

"Loss?"

"Right," I said. "How many of his patients have died during the procedure?"

"Died?" she moved back, astonished.

"That's right," I said, as puzzled now as she seemed to be. "I understand an average of one in two thousand is lost during a catheterization procedure?"

She gasped. "Dr. Narula has never lost anyone in a catheterization," she said flatly. "Not in twenty years."

"That's good," I smiled. "I did that death thing last week. I'm not ready to try it again."

The smile returned to her face. "Don't worry about Dr. Narula," she said softly. "You couldn't be in better hands. You'll be meeting him later today."

Dr. Salis left and I thought it was time to catch a quick nap. I was alone with my monitors. Our daughter, Karla, a student at the University of Central Florida, was driving Jo to Miami. I knew as soon as they checked into the motel, I'd be hearing from them. My body searched for a comfortable position on the bed.

A sharp shrill sound filled the room, sliced through sleep into my brain. I waited, hoping it would go away. It didn't. I pushed sleep aside and looked for the source of the noise. The phone, that's what it was, and I reached for the instrument.

"Hello."

"Honey, we made it," Jo's voice came over the line. "We're in the motel. We didn't have any trouble. Karla did a good job driving."

"That's good," I said, yawning to clear my mind. "You coming on over?"

"Soon as we can."

"Good, I would like you to be here when Dr. Narula arrives."

"I will be, honey," she promised. "I'll be there."

I placed the phone back in its cradle and rolled my body to face the door.

Flowers! Bouquets of beautiful flowers, all kinds, shapes, and colors, lined the shelf from the door across the wall.

"You are a popular man," a cocoa-skinned nurse with a Jamaican accent said entering the room. "All of these came for you while you were asleep."

"They're beautiful," I said just before she stuck a thermometer in my mouth.

She walked to the flowers, began studying them. "Would you like me to read the cards?"

"Please," I nodded.

"This beautiful Bird of Paradise arrangement is from Tom Brokaw, Bill Wheatley, and the NN staff," she said. "What's NN?"

"Nightly News," I answered. "Tom Brokaw is the anchor and Bill Wheatley is the Executive Producer. That's our prime news report."

She smiled, knowingly. "This next arrangement is from Jim Farley and the radio gang, and the next is from Howard Benedict, the President of the Canaveral Press Club, and the next is from Don Browne and the gang at the Miami Bureau, and the next is from . . .

She continued reading the names of friends and colleagues and I was pleased, and most grateful, for their thoughtfulness.

A white vampire came by for blood and my lunch was served, and before I had finished eating, Jo and Karla were there, oohing and ahhing over the flowers, and I felt settled in. The only thing irritating me was the fact that I hadn't had a shower since I fell on the beach.

"Nothing doing," said the nurse. "Dr. Narula will tell you when you can have a shower."

"When is he coming by?"

"Soon," she told me. "He's on the floor, he's making his rounds."

I felt a sense of anticipation, the knowing that someone

who would have a great deal to say about your future was about to arrive, a sort of sense of anticipating royalty.

A short while later the moment came. A bearded man with a beautiful blue turban on his head burst into the room with a broad, warm smile. "Hello, I'm Dr. Narula," he said. "And how are you feeling?"

"I think I'm fine," I said hoarsely, mesmerized by the headdress. I smiled to myself; Dr. Narula did not look his part. I half expected to see his elephant parked outside.

Just what I had imagined this world expert in cardiology would look like, I'm not really sure. I knew he was a countryman of Dr. Rajan's, but his turban had caught me off guard. I had not considered the fact he could be a member of the Sikh religious sect of northern India instead of being a Hindu like Dr. Rajan.

I was suddenly aware that my reaction had been formed by those prejudices most Americans freely carry with them and decided to cast them off.

Behind Dr. Narula, Dr. Salis was reviewing my condition and when she had finished, he began to ask questions of his own.

Minutes later, it was perfectly clear Dr. Narula was a man with an extraordinary grasp of any situation. He had the rare ability to correlate an enormous range of facts from various disciplines. And his wearing of a turban did not have a damn thing to do with the fact he was one of the most qualified experts in his field. I liked him right away.

Finished, he asked, "Do you have any questions?"

"What's the plan of attack?"

"We'll continue to monitor your condition for the next three days, and if there are no problems, if you continue to progress as well as you've been doing," he explained, "we'll do the catheterization Thursday, and the E.P. studies Friday. Anything else?"

"I would like to thank you for taking my case." I said sincerely. "I'm aware of how in demand you are, how many people need your help, and I want you to know I'm grateful."

"You're welcome." he said moving forward, and patting my hand. He turned with a smile for Jo, and as he walked from the room called back, "I'll see you tomorrow."

Instantly I knew I was in the right place and sighed with relief.

Later I learned how truly in demand Dr. Narula's services were. Not only did he maintain an office and practice in Cedars, and serve as a Clinical Professor of Cardiology at the University of Miami Medical School, he also maintained a worldwide practice.

He had authored three books on electrocardiography, published more than eighty papers, and was called on to lecture to scientific assemblies around the world.

Not only that but he was a pioneer in studying the electrophysiology of the heart and had developed a new technology in cardiac catheters for the treatment of patients with paroxysms (an intermittently rapid heart beat).

Dr. Narula had been developing an electrothermal catheter that heats up for two to three seconds to sever and cauterize heart muscle fibers that are out of synchronization with the heart's rhythm.

It would have been difficult to locate someone with better credentials. Dr. Onkar Narula was one doctor who had moved through medicine and beyond, and I was most grateful to have him.

For a small daily charge, the hospital moved a bed into the room for Jo. Three days passed as we watched television, and talked about what had to be done to put our house back in order.

Dr. Narula and the staff, monitored my every heartbeat, and their confidence slowly grew that my heart wouldn't have an encore of my "sudden death" performance.

Other than that one minor episode where my heart strung three PVCs, (premature ventricular contractions) together, it was performing like a champ.

Six days after I had fallen on the beach, Dr. Narula permitted me to take a shower, but with restrictions. They could remove my monitor leads but the I.V. had to stay in my arm.

The nurses wrapped the limb in plastic, and with it sticking out of the shower, I used my free hand to work in the shampoo and cover my body with refreshing, cleansing soap. Until you have been denied such routine hygiene, you cannot appreciate how pleasurable a shower can be.

That evening, my apprehension rose as I waited for the next day's catheterization procedure. Suddenly I was shocked to see a young lady at my bedside with a razor, shaving lather, and a pan of water.

"I'm here to shave you for your cath," she said.

"The hell you are," I snapped, disbelieving she could be serious.

The young lady stood there, frightened by my hostile reaction, wondering what to do next.

I offered her no way out. I was stunned. What shaving for a cath meant was the young lady would shave my groin area, including my genitalia, and being the father of two young women about her age, there was no way I was going to permit this.

She gathered her wits and managed a smile. "I do this all the time, Mr. Barbree," she said. "There's nothing to be embarrassed about."

"Oh, yeah?" I barked. "I'll let you shave my genitals if you will let me shave yours."

Her face blushed. She too was embarrassed.

"Do we have a deal?" I questioned.

"No," she protested, "of course not."

"What the hell is wrong with this place," I protested. "Why don't they have a man come around to do this?" I shouted. "When I had a catheterization in Gainesville, they sent a man."

"Please, Mr. Barbree," she pleaded. "This is my job. I'm a student," she explained. "I need the money."

Jo walked to the bed, laughing. "Oh, Jay," she scolded. "Don't be so modest. Let her do her job."

"You wanta' have your genitals shaved by a college student, a male college student?" I snapped back at my wife.

"No," Jo laughed louder, going through the door. "I'm leaving, getting outta' Dodge."

"Coward," I yelled, turning my attention back to the young lady. "I suggest you follow her, Miss."

The young lady stood there, puzzled, wondering what to do next, but she didn't have to wonder long.

Two nurses—big, big nurses burst through the door and surrounded my bed, both with penetrating stares that said without words they would tolerate no bullshit.

"What's the problem, Mr. Barbree?" the one who had visible imprints of football cleats on her forehead asked.

"I want a man to shave me," I said timidly.

"Nonsense," King Kong of nurses bellowed, reaching for the sheets as the other burly, nurse held my limbs. "We don't have any male nurses on this floor, Mr. Barbree, and we are not the least bit interested in what you have between your legs," she said sternly, joining her partner in the task of removing my underwear.

Suddenly, and without choice, my naked body was exposed, and the former gridiron pros held me firm as the young lady began her work.

I gave up. I was outnumbered and deserted by my faithful partner. Hell, I grinned to myself. Old faithful Jo was, without question, the one who sent those two linebackers to rescue the young lady.

I transferred my thoughts elsewhere and ignored the scrapings of the razor, ignored the small talk, especially ignored the snickers.

Morning found us in the Cardiac Catheterization Laboratory deep within the test facilities that were the Cedars Medical Center.

I had been given my "happy shot" in my room and a warm and gentle young lady with a touch of Spanish in her voice was busy connecting a bottle of fluid to my I.V. to feed, if necessary, life-saving medications directly into my bloodstream.

The cardiac catheterization is not surgery, but the nurses and technicians, and Dr. Narula himself, wore surgical masks and gowns to help keep the equipment sterile.

Another nurse was busy scrubbing my right groin where the catheter would be inserted. Sterile towels and a sheet was placed around the area while a technician loaded film into the x-ray camera.

It was the technician's job to get all the equipment ready and during "small talk" I learned he was studying to become a priest.

"Hope we don't need your services," I said.

"Not today," Dr. Narula laughed, as he moved to make a small incision in the skin to locate the desired artery.

The groin had been numbed with a local anesthetic similar to the novocaine used by dentists. There was a slight sting, but no pain, and once the artery had been located, he placed a large needle in it to serve as a sheath to guide each catheter through the vessel.

I had been strapped to a table-like bed that could move from side to side under a rotating camera, and it was time for me to relax, to watch the overhead television monitors that Dr. Narula would use to trace the catheters into my heart.

I reassured myself these people knew what they were doing. I watched as Dr. Narula snaked the first of the catheters through my leg, into the chest area where the tube moved into my heart. The picture gave me the feeling it was happening to someone else. It was difficult for me to understand the catheter was in my body, not in another person's, that person's body displayed on the television screen.

I reasoned my mind was playing this trick on me because there was no pain. No discomfort. Blood vessels do not have pain fibers, and the only part of the procedure I felt was when the dye was injected through the catheter into my heart. There was a sudden warmth, a sensation like hot water flushing through my chest. It passed quickly and we all watched the blood flow through some of my heart's coronary arteries.

Of course, I didn't know if what we saw was good or bad, but I was certain I had detected disappointment in Dr. Narula's eyes.

When the procedure was over, and I had been wheeled back to my room, I began to wonder about what Dr. Narula had seen. I tried to be patient.

I knew the film had to be developed first, then Dr.

Narula had to study it, make precise measurements. He had promised to see me in the afternoon, and until then, there was really nothing to do but wait and try to eat breakfast lying flat on my back.

The day passed slowly. I was restricted to bed rest, not permitted to move my right leg. It was important that the groin not be bent so that a good seal could form in the incision where the catheters were inserted.

Jo and I watched TV, made small talk, but we both were anxious to know the results of the test.

It came in mid-afternoon when a sober Dr. Narula entered the room. He didn't waste time. "We have problems."

"Bad problems?" my heart leaped into my throat.

"Difficult problems, but manageable," he said firmly. "Your coronary artery disease has progressed, and you have three new lesions."

"What do I have now, six?"

"That's about right," he nodded in the affirmative. "The original lesions have become worse and you have the new ones."

"What's the answer? The bypass?"

"Well, not ideally," he said, beginning a lengthy explanation. "Because of your young age, and the natural progression of coronary artery disease with time, I would like to defer surgery as long as possible so that we do not have to operate on you a second time."

The thunderbolt impact of that statement stunned me, made me feel my luck had deserted me. In the bargain it had not simply walked out the door, it had run, and I knew enough about coronary artery disease to know the depth of my problem.

The coronary arteries supply the heart with life-sustaining blood. If they are clogged, if they shut down, then the result is a heart attack, killing the part of the organ starved for blood.

Dr. Narula continued to explain my predicament, drawing pictures of the plaque that had formed on the coronary artery walls, calling attention to the percentage each one was closed.

He especially dwelled on one lesion at the top of my coronaries, one that appeared eighty percent closed, restricting blood flow to the branches of the arteries themselves.

You didn't have to be a rocket scientist to understand if the plaque in the lesion was permitted to grow, it would shut off the blood flow to most of my heart and the result would be almost certain death.

Dr. Narula went on to explain that neither the coronary bypass operation nor the "balloon" angioplasty procedure were ideal choices to fix my problem.

My coronaries were being eaten alive by plaque forming on their walls and any effort to reopen them with angioplasty, a catheter with a balloon on the tip, would be risky.

In the procedure, the balloon is pushed inside the lesion and then inflated and deflated for several seconds to try to flatten the buildup of plaque against the artery wall. When it works, this widens the artery, and good blood flow returns. But when there are two, three, or more lesions in a row on the same artery the physician must try to open each lesion, multiplying the risks. Sometimes the plaque is crushed and the artery's wall collapses. The vessel refuses to stay open and a heart attack follows. Immediate bypass surgery is needed to keep the patient alive.

The Barbree curse had raised its ugly head. My chances of celebrating more than one or two more birthdays were slim and none, and I spent the evening trying to digest all I'd been told.

Jo, bless her, tried to be cheerful, but we both knew I was in deep trouble and each of us tried to conjure up a solution.

What we both understood without discussing it was that the situation must be kept between us, kept from the rest of the family, kept from friends, but more importantly, kept from NBC News.

It wasn't that the company could not be trusted, but there were financial situations to be considered, and after twenty-nine years with the network, I wanted to return to work if possible, wanted another shot at a normal life even though it appeared that my life expectancy could be measured on a twelve-month calendar.

For the moment, though, staying alive was *the*, and only, issue.

Until this moment I had been pleased to let the doctors worry about my condition. Oh, I had been trying to help by watching my diet, and jogging, staying in shape. But now it was clear I must get into the act. If I was to survive more than one or two years, I had to take responsibility for my own health. I had to start digging for answers. After all, that's what I did for a living, looked for answers in mountains of research, and this time, the mountain I must climb would be my last if I didn't find a path down the other side.

I slept little that night, but I wasn't all that tired when they came for me the next morning for a trip to another lab with catheters. This time the catheters were smaller and they had a different mission.

I was readied to undergo what is called baseline electrophysiological studies. What that meant was Dr. Narula wanted to see if he could entice my heart to leap into ventricular tachycardia (sudden death) by performing electrical stimulation using a system similar to a pacemaker.

I spent three hours on the table with wires running through the catheters into my heart. Dr. Narula was searching for something wrong with my heart's electrical system. He explained that faulty fibers, which sometime act like transmitting wires, send the wrong signals to the heart. These may be abnormally present from birth, or may result from a previous heart attack with muscle damage and scar tissue formation. This may cause the heart to beat too fast and develop ventricular tachycardia, or ventricular fibrillation.

In a normal heart, there is a safety mechanism that prevents these natural "wires" from transmitting incorrect messages, and in my case, my luck returned—my safety mechanism was intact. Shock pattern after shock pattern failed to break my heart's normal rhythm. It performed like a champ. Dr. Narula could not make it miss a beat.

The test showed that my "sudden death" was, in all probability, brought on by lack of blood flow through the clogged coronary arteries, and Dr. Narula concluded that I would have never experienced "sudden death" if I had not been jogging, and had not pushed my body to total exhaustion.

The baseline electrophysiological studies also served another purpose. They helped Dr. Narula prescribe the precise medications needed for my condition, and during my remaining stay in the hospital, he monitored my response to the medicines.

Dr. Narula told me the good news was that my heart itself had not been damaged, there had been no heart attack, and the organ itself was in good shape. But the bad news was the coronary arteries, the heart's only source for life-giving blood, were greatly diseased.

He told me there were two ways I could get myself into another life-threatening situation. One, if I was foolish enough to totally exhaust myself again, or two, if I permitted any of the lesions in my coronary arteries to progress to complete closure.

The first threat I could control. The second would require a total commitment to learning how I could continue to live, and the total dedication and disciplines necessary to put those lessons learned into practice.

The electrophysiological studies were better than we had hoped, and with a strong heart muscle, and with my tailor-made medication program prescribed and tested by Dr. Narula, there was suddenly confidence my heart disease could be managed.

But because the cardiac catheterization had painted such a gloomy picture of multiple lesions closing my coronary arteries, Dr. Narula decided on one more test. A thallium stress test, which is a tread mill stress test procedure in which radioactive material is used to take pictures which show the amount of blood flowing through the heart.

I passed this one with ease, and the picture brightened even more. Dr. Narula said he would send my catheterization films to centers specializing in balloon angioplasty in order to confirm his decision that the balloon dilation procedure was not an ideal option for me. We were convinced we had a grip on my condition. With ample blood flow to my heart muscle, and with my strengthened *will* to take care of myself, suddenly a normal life appeared possible.

A smile returned to Jo's face. We had a shot at beating the odds. We were ready to do battle with my heart disease.

After nearly two weeks at Cedars Medical Center, what I had come to think of as the umbilical cords, thin and thick, tiny and powerful, were removed so that I was no longer symbiotic with machinery, drugs, pressures, electricity and all the other confining tools of medicine. At first they had given me confidence. While I had lain in my hospital bed, they were my link to continued life. They were watchdogs. Angels. Call them what you will; they were monitors and the systems needed to sound a strident alarm if "sudden death" came to me again, if any other physiological component showed even the signs of failure.

Even if I did not know something was wrong, the monitors would tell all, instantly, to the doctors and nurses and they would rush to my aid. But there was not a flutter, a tweak, a slip, a hesitation in the body, and all the tests were done. After nearly two weeks, I was glad to see them go. I had begun to weary of pinioned imprisonment.

I was ready to go home.

Jo was ecstatic at the prospects of getting my heart disease under control, of my getting a new lease on life, and minutes later she was driving us up Florida's Turnpike, headed for what we called "The Barbree Coast," which we jokingly had named our home on the ocean. In little more than three hours, we were there, walking on the beach.

I took an extra large gulp of salt air and waved at the seagulls and the pelicans, noticing that even the sandpipers seemed to sprint about the sand with more life. It was good to be alive, to be home. I looked at the horizon, wondered at how that far edge of earth fell away in its spectacular curve, wondered if my coronary artery disease would permit me to see that splendid view from space.

The thought caused me to turn my head to the left, to stare at the mighty gantries and towers of Cape Canaveral from which the great rockets rise on columns of flame to reach the vacuum high above; the same launch pads for the historical and contemporary machines I had covered and broadcast and written about for decades. I was suddenly aware all the thrills were still there, only better.

I still wanted to be on the Journalist-in-Space flight. Maybe more now than ever. As I stood there, surrounded by life, I looked around at the rich green of the flora from Jo's landscaping efforts, and I was pleased to see the four coconut palms I had planted before my fall on the beach.

Few dared to attempt to grow coconut trees as far north as Cocoa Beach, but not me. The coconut tree's long, flowing fronds are my favorite tropical foliage. It is nature's creation that tells you you are on that part of the earth where the temperature never reaches freezing.

In a way, the now-thriving coconut trees were symbolic of my own condition. We both were full of life, eager to grow, to live despite our precarious choice of environments and we could if only we were given proper care. This, I told myself, was the beginning of my second life.

FIFTEEN

"Starting Over"

Daylight came alive with Florida's brilliant sunshine, with a red bird prancing and singing on one of the limbs of the magnolia tree outside our bedroom window. I almost leapt from the bed. I was so eager to pick up my life, to take control of my health, to understand what had to be done for me to live.

Although I have long been in favor of preventive medicine, I would soon learn I had taken on a heavy chore. Man had spent centuries trying to cope with heart disease, and here I was trying to learn how to deal with man's number one killer with a short-term effort.

Despite this shortcoming, I spent the next few weeks researching, reading everything I could get my hands on dealing with heart disease, and being a reporter, my telephone calls were accepted by some of the leading authorities on the subject in the world.

Dr. Narula had sent me home with one major objective in mind. Keep track of the growth of my coronary artery disease. Do not permit it to shut down the vital blood supply to my heart.

To accomplish this, Dr. Narula felt we must find a way to reduce my overall blood cholesterol to 150, and to develop an exercise program that would keep my heart and body in top shape while not exhausting myself to the point where I could again trigger "sudden death."

An average, or below average blood pressure was also important, and, of course, no smoking.

But, thankfully, smoking was no longer a battle for me. I had defeated the habit in the late 1970s, during the days when Jimmy Carter was President, and when I drew the assignment to cover the President when he was home in Plains, Georgia for Christmas or summer vacation.

Most reporters smoked in the 1950s and 1960s and even though we knew better in the 1970s, it was next to impossible for most of us to give up the filthy weed.

For many of us, the President's brother, Billy, was our good-time hero, our leader on the softball field as we took on the team fielded by the President, his staff, and Secret Service.

Billy was always good for a laugh because he was never without a cigarette in one hand and a beer in the other, not even during the sunup hours. Billy could be found at our motel, at the breakfast round table, drinking beer and puffing a cigarette while we tried to down eggs, grits, hash browns, pancakes, toast, or cereal.

"You folks don't know what's good," Billy would pontificate as he drank the now defunct Billy Beer and puffed on the weed.

We would all laugh and join him later for the softball game where by the end of the contest he was seldom standing.

One day when I was umpire, Billy could hardly roll the ball over the plate, let alone pitch it there. It reached the point where I had to call anything he got over the plate a strike, and later President Carter, whose team beat Billy's easily, said, "We had the best team, but Billy had the umpire."

The President was correct, of course. Many of us felt sorry for Billy and his problem with alcohol and cigarettes. Most of us knew he was a good man, a true product of a small town and easy living and he had to live everyday with the fact he was "First Brother."

Often we heard Billy say he wished Jimmy didn't have that "Job," as he would call it, but Jimmy did, and because of it, Billy could no longer be just one of the boys at the local service station.

Billy would later give up drinking and smoking, taking the cure, but in the end cancer got him as it did his father and sisters.

A mutual friend, Clarence Gibbons, a cameraman for CBS News, was one of Billy's pallbearers, and Clarence told me how Billy was that small town boy to the end, how he wanted to be buried in his Tom T. Hall T-shirt beneath the dress shirt and suit he only wore when necessary.

We who knew him loved Billy Carter. We loved him because he was an honest man, not a phoney. If he liked you, you knew it. If he didn't, you knew that too.

There was *no* politician in Billy Carter, and we understood him. We understood that in Billy's world drinking beer was a password. We understood that once upon a time it was cool to smoke. Once upon a time everyone smoked, and teens in those years all worked hard at learning to inhale.

But in the 1990s, smoking definitely is not cool. There is no longer any question that nicotine is as addictive as heroin and cocaine. It kills more than 300,000 people every year, far more than heroin and cocaine and all hard drugs, and it killed a man I dearly loved.

My father-in-law Jack Reisinger died from lung cancer due to smoking, and it was one of the worst deaths a person could endure. Lungs rotting inside of an otherwise healthy body, nurses trying to keep the throat clear, trying to kill the pain.

We have all lost friends and family to the legal poison named nicotine, and I was glad with my tough fight against heart disease ahead that my battle with nicotine had already been won.

For the first step of the seven-step-plan, they thought it would be best for me to get my diet house in order.

What we were learning from the experts in the field suggested it wasn't enough to follow the American Heart Association's recommendation of cutting fat intake to about thirty-percent of total calories, ten-percent or less was what was really needed to get results.

A panel of health and nutrition experts at the National

Research Council was recommending that a person should eat five or more servings of fruits and vegetables, and six or more helpings of breads, cereals and legumes every day.

The experts added a person should only eat moderate amounts of protein and maintain an adequate calcium intake.

This advice was consistent with Nathan Pritikin's diet, a diet with a superb track record for fighting coronary artery disease and I set out to learn how best to secure such a diet, and put it on my table.

Step two of the program was to be exercise, a tailor-made exercise program to fit my situation.

What I was learning from current research was that only about eight-percent of adults in this country were getting adequate exercise. What I also learned was about twenty-minutes of aerobic exercise (sustained walking, running, cycling) three times each week is all that was needed to keep fit.

According to the experts, aerobic exercise helps supply the heart muscle with increased oxygen and improves muscle tone and mass, strengthening the heart. There is also evidence it raises HDL levels (the good cholesterol needed to keep your arteries clean), and aerobic exercise helps keep body weight down.

Of course, it was my jogging that permitted me to push myself to total exhaustion and bring on "sudden death." Doctors Narula and Rajan wanted none of that, and they gave me limits in which I could increase my heart rate. It was decided my exercise program would be limited to a stretching and brisk walking agenda.

For step number three we monitored my blood pressure closely to make sure the medications and diet kept it below normal, and for step number four we tackled the all-important cholesterol problem. We had one objective, get the total cholesterol down to 150, and increase the HDL cholesterol (the good stuff).

There was good reason behind the thinking of Doctors Narula and Rajan to make such an assault on my cholesterol levels because experts had learned that in people with inherited coronary disease the liver routes excess cholesterol back to the bloodstream where it could get picked up by body tissues and stored.

It was also clear that my liver, as it does in most people, was producing eighty-percent of the cholesterol in my body. With diet and exercise I hoped to reduce my cholesterol levels through twenty-percent.

Dr. Narula put me on medication to lower the cholesterol levels and we were off and running.

Steps number five, six, and seven of the program took us beyond intervention into revitalizing the body with medications and foods and exercises. It also took us into the use of the mind.

First of all in this part of the program, it was important that I retained the *WILL* to live, that my goals were what they had always been, that my dignity, my worth was intact.

Step number six was simple: Don't worry, be happy.

Psychological stress did in fact affect heart disease. Not in the tradition of the stressful job, but through hostility and mistrust.

Based on animal studies, researchers had identified biochemicals released during stress that seem to contribute to arterial injuries and cause the formation of plaque on artery walls. And this was not just evident in people with the classic Type A personality who are at risk for a heart attack. Some investigators say that anyone who exhibits chronic hostility and mistrust produces the stress response that can lead to coronary problems.

This hit closer to home than I cared to admit. All one has to do is be cut off in traffic a couple of times and you quickly learn how much of a pacifist you really are.

The program we had selected seemed simple enough. Cut cholesterol levels to the bone, eat a fat-free diet, stay trim by exercising regularly, and of course don't smoke, and leave your hostility and mistrust at home.

Despite my health objectives as I eased back into my job, it was clear to me I had to downplay my heart disease, not only because of having to compete with younger reporters for my livelihood, but because I was a finalist in the Journalist-in-Space project. As long as there was any hope that I could make the flight, I wanted to remain in the running.

I had received a certificate from The Association of Schools of Journalism and Mass Communication recognizing me as a national finalist in the project, and, in an accompanying letter, the ASJMC (The ASJMC was the organization selected by NASA to select finalists for the Journalist-In-Space,) informed me that the Journalist-In-Space Project was officially on "hold" until NASA recovered from the Challenger accident. The letter went on to state that once NASA had decided it was safe to fly civilians, the Teacher-in-Space would be the first to go, with the Journalist scheduled next.

That gave me some extra time and kept me in the contest. With the Journalist-In-Space on hold, I reasoned, I would have time to take care of my coronary artery disease problem and I would still have a shot at making the flight.

Not long after I got back to work I was the guest on a radio affiliate's call-in talk show, I was answering questions about the Journalist-In-Space project when this man called in and said bluntly, "I hope Walter Cronkite gets the ride, he deserves it."

"Why does he deserve it, sir?" I asked.

"Because he's Walter Cronkite," the man said, obviously amazed I would even ask. "He's earned it," the man continued. "He's Walter Cronkite."

"I understand Walter is a big *"STAR,"* I said, starting to steam "but why has he earned it anymore than I have or other reporters who have covered many more space missions than Cronkite?"

"Because he is Walter Cronkite," the impatient caller said. "He's Cronkite and you and those other guys are nothing."

I bit my lip. My temper was on "high boil" again, and Jim Burns, the host of the show, knew it was time to go to a commercial. The caller had hit a raw spot in my projected replanning of my "hot tempered" psyche. I seethed, of course, we other finalists had seen more than one gleaming, capped-tooth idiot on TV express their opinion that they hoped Cronkite was chosen because, in their opinion, he had *earned* the ride.

Despite wanting to remain calm, my questions rose to the surface. Where is it etched in granite that *"STARS"* deserve all of life's blessings? Where is it etched in granite that none of the grunts in the trenches deserve a break?

Without question Walter Cronkite was a beloved news anchor who was paid millions of dollars, and still is paid a reported million dollars a year in retirement.

He showed up to cover the early manned space flights and the landings on the moon a couple of days before each event. He had hundreds of researchers and staff holding his hand, but what about the reporters who spent every day of their lives covering space flight? The reporters like the late Mary Bubb, who was there to write about the most insignificant launch as well as the historic missions.

For more than thirty years Mary Bubb wrote for the wire services and for magazines, often the only reporter there to ask questions after each launch, and she did it before women were freely admitted into the male-dominated profession of journalism.

Devotion? Hell, Mary Bubb invented the word, and when she died, her life's work was so well admired, some NASA workers and reporters surreptitiously spread her ashes around the space center's press site and launch pads where astronauts stepped into orbit and traveled to the moon.

Mary Bubb was one who paid her dues, who *earned* the right to be the first Journalist-in-Space, and she left few worldly things behind. She was *not* a millionaire star of our profession. Good Lord! She barely kept body and soul together, but she was a cornerstone of journalism's foundation.

And when it comes to paying dues, how about the AP's Howard Benedict. He covered space from 1959 to 1990 before retiring to serve as the Executive Director of the Mercury Seven Foundation.

Of course, there are many more unknown journalists who keep the profession on a straight course for minimum pay. Don't they deserve a little recognition for their devotion and unceasing efforts?

I believe they do. I believe it is fair and just, and for those with their quick and shallow opinions, I say, "It is not written in stone that the big hog gets all the corn." There's gotta' be a few grains left for the rest of us.

Anyway, I finally calmed down, realized the caller was just expressing his damned opinion, and got back to work on the task of trying to live less stressfully if not less busily for as I picked up my life and started over, if I wasn't researching the latest facts and cures for heart disease, I was actively covering NASA's recovery from the Challenger accident.

The press is kept corralled on a mound of earth in the shadow of the Kennedy Space Center's giant Vehicle Assembly Building, three to four miles from the two space shuttle launch pads.

Each of the networks, wires services, and other news organizations are leased plots of land on the top of the mound where we park trailers, or in the case of the networks, where we put up our own building equipped with offices and studios.

In the adjacent large geodesic dome, the NASA Public Affairs staff operates an information center for working reporters.

The press site is a workable arrangement for both press and NASA, and it offers a closed community that is mostly business but is not without its fun.

When the ABC News building was first under construction, the builder made one small error. He constructed the facility facing away from the launch pad. The red-faced network had to bring in two giant cranes to turn the building around so their cameras and reporters could see the space shuttles thundering into the sky.

And there was the time some NBC people thought it would be a good idea to leave the press mound for a closer view of a huge Saturn-V moon rocket on display near the giant Vehicle Assembly Building. Of course, they were arrested for not having proper badges but the NBC people knew what to do. They called their boss. The network executive and his staff went to their rescue only to be arrested

themselves. Finally, someone got the idea they should call a
NASA press escort and the problem was resolved.

On another day an out-of-town reporter stepped out of
his trailer and assumed a fifteen-foot alligator that had
crawled out of the nearby swamp was tame. He would later
say he never knew 'gators, or he, could run so fast.

Another newspaper type wasn't fast enough. Portable
toilets are stationed in rows along the press mound, and
when the portable structures were ordered hauled away to
make room for fresher ones, the horrified reporter's fading
screams could not be heard over the noise of the crane-outfit-
ted-truck driving off the mound.

Dangers on the famed press site are not limited to manmade structures or wildlife. The mound has its pranksters,
and none are more devilish than the AP's Harry Rosenthal.

During one shuttle mission when noted broadcaster Jim
Slade was on the air live for the Mutual Radio Network,
staring at the launch pad through a large window at the end
of his trailer, Rosenthal decided to show him a cartoon he
had cut out of a publication.

Slade violated a cardinal rule of broadcasting; never
permit yourself to be distracted while on the air live. All too
often people go out of their way to break you up on the air,
but they can only get away with it if you pay them notice.

Rosenthal held the cartoon flat against Slade's studio
window and while the words continued to roll smoothly
from his lips, Jim studied the drawing of Moses standing at
the foot of the mountain holding the tablets with God's Ten
Commandments.

One of Moses' followers says: "Let me get this straight.
You want us to cut the heads off of our penises?"

The words ceased coming from Slade's mouth. He
slumped across his broadcast table, laughing hysterically.

Such events were part of my daily fare, and it has long
been established that laughter is good for the soul. Only a
few weeks passed before I felt like I was back in the groove,
putting "sudden death" behind me.

And, of course, I began to play a few pranks myself.

As the reporter who broke the cause of the Challenger
blowup, and as one of a handful of journalists who had cov-

ered NASA for three decades, I often found my actions being watched by reporters new to the space beat.

It was difficult for a new reporter who had been sent in to cover NASA's recovery from the Challenger disaster to develop independent sources, and most were left standing in the news center, waiting for official handouts.

The result was, any time I went through the dome and into one of the Public Affairs people's offices, I found my visit being watched closely.

The most sought-after NASA spokesman was the Chief of Information and the voice of launch control, Hugh Harris.

The facts are that although Hugh Harris, now a Deputy Director, Dick Young, now Chief of Information, and the boss himself, Director of Public Affairs Chuck Hollinshead are cut from the cloth of nice people, the bottom line is that they are professionals. They are there to serve NASA's interests and they never favor one reporter over the other. They try to give everyone an even break.

Any time I had a reason to visit Hugh's office was generally to check past facts, and this one particular morning the dome was jammed with reporters waiting for a crucial NASA announcement on when the agency hoped to resume its shuttle flights.

After spending a few moments behind closed doors with Mr. Harris, I opened his office door and within ear shot of most of the reporters suspiciously watching me, I yelled, "Thanks, Hugh," and broke into a run through the crowd and out of the dome.

As I went through the door I could hear the frenzied yells over my shoulder, "What'd he tell you?"

"Hey, Barbree, what's happening?"

"He's got something," another called out.

As I ran into the NBC building to hide, NASA folks were set upon by reporters demanding to know what I knew, what I'd been told. Few believed Hugh Harris and his staff when they assured them I had been told nothing more than they had been told.

It felt good to laugh, not to take life so seriously, especially since I have been on the receiving end of making a fool out of myself many times.

It is not at all unusual to brush shoulders with celebrities around the press site. Jimmy Stewart and wife have been there along with Robert Redford, Dennis Quaid, John Denver, and many others, and often they will get underfoot, get in the way during the critical moments of reporting a lift-off.

I will never forget one shuttle launch when I was on the air live only to have three women walk in front of my studio window and block my view of the shuttle.

Quickly, I pounded an angry fist on the glass, demanding with an arm gesture that they move. They did, graciously.

The following morning when I picked up the local newspaper, I stared at a front page photograph of Carol Burnett, her daughter, and a press spokesperson standing on the NBC front porch, viewing the launch. My myopic intensity of the moment kept me from recognizing one of my favorite entertainers, but later, at Disney World, I had the opportunity to apologize to Ms. Burnett.

In spite of the embarrassing moments, the childlike pranks, and the competitive intensity of the assignments, it was my job that restored me to what seemed a normal life.

In fact getting back to work is the therapy recommended by many physicians, and late in the summer of '87, I was functioning in my job as if nothing happened.

My cholesterol was down where the doctors wanted it, along with my weight, and my exercise program was right on target as well as my blood pressure. The only items not under control were attitude, temperament, hostility, and most of all heredity, the things that couldn't be measured.

One day I sat in the NBC building, studying the shuttle launch pads, wondering if they would ever again be active, but, somewhere beneath these focused thoughts was the nagging question of what had caused my "sudden death" on the beach. During this period I was more concerned with the wear and tear of stress and hostility, in addition to the unhealthy diet and lack of exercise that went along with the day-in and day-out news coverage.

Producer Art Lord, a friend for many years, had a saying about working in the pressure-cooker world of TV news: "Short fuse, short memory."

That pretty well summed it up. The pressure of a deadline often replaces the social niceties with screams and shots. But after the job is done, after the report is on the air, the friendly attitudes reemerges, and life is pleasant. We are all once again friends. Hostility is put back in its box where it stays until it is again released by the key of stress.

But the questions bothering me were how many years of my life was I surrendering to compete in the high-pressure world of news coverage? How many years was I surrendering to my classic type-A personality? To my inherited hostility?

Researchers have identified biochemicals released during hostility that seem to contribute to arterial injuries and set the stage for the formation of plaque in the arteries. Investigators like Dr. Robert Eliot, Director of the Cardiovascular Institute at Swedish Medical Center in Denver, say anyone who exhibits chronic hostility and cynical mistrust produces the stress that can lead to heart problems.

Blood pressure, cholesterol, exercise, diet, things that could be measured directly I had under control. But attitude, hostility were another kettle of fish.

Oh, I've often reminded myself of the cute little sayings like rule number one: Don't sweat the small stuff. Rule number two: It's all small stuff. And my favorite: They can't get your goat if they don't know where he's tied.

All of these sayings make perfect sense. Anyone with half a brain should agree with them. Then, what the hell happens when someone cuts you off in traffic? What happens when someone jumps ahead of you in line? Or blocks the highway?

Some people let it roll off them like water rolling off a duck's back. It simply doesn't bother them. But not me, and not millions of others.

I realize hostility, a classic type-A personality, is an inherited trait. But what can you do about it?

I remember in school how my sister Jean was always getting in fights to protect me and my sister Billie.

Hardly a day passed we didn't hear some kids on the playground yelling, "Fight, fight," and many times when we got to the scene we would see feet, arms, and red hair flying. Jean *was* in the middle.

The kids used to sing a little song to get her goat. They would point an accusing finger at her and sing, "Red headed woodpecker sitting on a log. She fell off and turned to a frog."

It's funny to us today, but not then. We stuck together, and if you picked a fight with one, you'd have us all to whip.

The way we respond to taunts, rudeness, and ignorance plays a significant role in the growth of heart disease.

Dr. Robert Eliot says that's because we are living in the bodies of our cavemen ancestors in a world they never thought was possible.

Dr. Eliot reports our brains and bodies have been programmed from prehistoric time to release hormones like adrenalin—even cholesterol—to speed reaction to danger, what we perceive as a threat, or stress.

"While cavemen may have fought a saber-tooth tiger a couple times in a lifetime," Dr. Eliot said, "many people now are fighting tigers many times a day."

Studies by Eliot show that an abundance of stress hormones released into the bloodstream by the brain causes lesions in the heart and changes in blood vessel walls.

Studies of Navy pilots show cholesterol levels are highest among those landing planes on aircraft carriers, though all had similar diets.

Experts say most doctors treating heart disease don't consider the role of the brain, and Dr. Eliot said, "It's like mopping water off the floor without turning off the faucet."

Some research suggest behavior modification can help, but the question I was still asking was how?

Throughout NASA's recovery from the Challenger accident and return to space flight, as well as my own recovery from "sudden death" on the beach, I was attempting to change my attitude, to get my hostility under control through simple faith.

One thing that helped me, and seemed to help a colleague, was my own changing perspective on life itself.

This colleague (if I named him you would know him) was always stressed out before he had to do a live report on television. He was convinced what he was about to do was the most important thing in the world, and he was equally convinced that he was going to mess up. At times he worried so much he would throw up before going on the air.

One day a short while after my hospitalization I stood there watching him sweat, waiting for the camera to come alive, and the following thought occured to me. "Buddy, it's only television," I told him. "It's not open-heart surgery."

He grinned. You could see his muscles relax, and since that day, it's been easier for my colleague; not a laid-back performance, but easier.

Without question my words helped me also. Today, I'm as relaxed going live on television as I am sitting in my own home. In fact, like most people who try to reform their own lives I can't resist commenting to those people who get uptight over the most trivial things. My wife for example, has a fit over hanging a crooked picture in my studio or placing furniture in unauthorized places about the house.

Yes I was more calm than I used to be. The truth is the farther along in my recovery I got, the more I was getting control of controlled situations. It was the unexpected which continued to light my short fuse.

In order to deal with it I found myself reaching back to my roots not relying entirely on facts but turning more and more towards faith.

SIXTEEN

"Faith"

The beautiful lady stood ghostlike at the foot of the bed, smiling. Her image grew and faded in clarity, illuminating the dark night. In her dream-like state, my mother stared through what had been sleep, wondering if she was dreaming, yet more sure with each passing moment she was awake.

It was still more than two hours before dawn, and as my mother's mind cleared she realized the beautiful lady was a stranger, not a family member, not a neighbor, but a friend. There was no reason to be afraid, to cry out for help.

My mother raised up in bed and started to speak but instantly she knew words were unnecessary. She returned the smile and waited, wondered who the beautiful lady could be.

"He is with us," the lady said softly. "He is not where you put him," she added as her image began to fade.

Tears filled my mother's eyes as she stretched a hand toward the disappearing lady, hearing her say, "Be in peace," before she was gone.

My mother slumped back on her bed, tears flowing down her face, tears of peace and relief.

For weeks my mother had been carrying a heavy burden. One of my brothers, born earlier than I, had stepped on a rusty nail, and 1925 country doctors knew little about treating tetanus. It was simply called "lockjaw," and death was certain.

My brother, named Willie Lee, was only eleven years old and he died in my parents' arms. After burial, my mother's grief held her close to the cemetery, especially during thunderstorms. Willie Lee had been afraid of lightning and during a storm she would go and sit on his grave, a mother protecting her child.

The family minister had tried to console her, as had my father and eldest sister, Lois. But nothing worked, nothing relieved her grief, lifted her burden until the beautiful lady stood at the foot of her bed. It was a story every member of the family knew, and as I was just a child its truthfulness was never questioned by me.

I grew up in a Christian home and, as most who did, I believed in God, in Heaven, and in Hell, and generally accepted the teachings of the Bible. It would be years before I would begin questioning this faith.

I suppose I began to wonder about a higher authority when I became a reporter, when the first tool of my trade was the use of the question. Most of the stories I was assigned to cover were in the world of science, and I found it easier not to believe than to believe. I did not argue when I heard scientists and colleagues refer to the Bible as a fable.

Wiser men than I warned there were two subjects to avoid: politics and religion. I found myself heeding this advice.

I've often thought about my mother's story of the beautiful lady at the foot of my parents' bed and I suppose today I would be more inclined to believe the lady was born out of my mother's grief than I am inclined to believe she actually appeared. Still I wonder.

Before I dropped dead jogging, I had firm ideas about the death penalty, and many other social and political axioms. In fact, there were few things in life in which I did not have a firm opinion.

After my experience with death, and when my mind cleared, I found myself no longer so positive, no longer believing in the death penalty, willing to leave that judgement and other judgements to God Himself, a God I was and am sure is there.

What I am not sure of after "sudden death" is, is God the God of Christians? Or is He the God of the Hindus? Perhaps He is the God of the Moslems? Could it be so simple that He is the God of all people? After my experience, one thing is certain. I can only wonder, can only question.

There is no authoritarian answer. There are so many answers that man can never hope to know it all, to come close to understanding the wonders of the heavens, the secrets of the universe and the creation.

One of my favorite questions for scientists when they start explaining the "big bang" theory that created the universe, is where did the matter, the material come from for the "big bang?"

Not long after my "death," during one of the briefings for the launch of the large Hubble Space Telescope, I asked a panel of the nation's top scientists that question. The scientists agreed the question was without answer, but the President of the American Astronomical Society, Dr. John Bachall of Princeton University, came up to me and requested that I ask him the question when it was the astronomers' turn.

I did, and Dr. Bachall explained that his wife was a professor of astronomy at Princeton. He said that he had asked her what she told her students when they asked the same question, she took him through a lengthy, detailed scientific theory. But he felt he could boil the answer down to one word.

We all waited for *the* word. Dr. Bachall stared at me. It was clear he wanted me to be his straight man, and I asked, "And, what is that one word, Doctor?"

"Foreplay."

The news conference roared with laughter. We tend to dismiss many unknowns in the most convenient manner, and humor is an easy tool of convenience.

I suppose I first began thinking seriously about the unknown, the possibility of something beyond death when our son, Scott, was born five weeks premature. His tiny lungs had not matured and he developed Hyaline Membrane Disease. We were hoping against hope that he would make it, that he would live, but at the moment he died I was at a friend's house, and when that moment took place, I knew it. Something swept over me, telling me to drive quickly to the hospital, to my wife's bedside.

I drove as quickly as I could and within ten minutes I was in her room, seeing the tears roll down her face, listening to the Doctor tell her that Scott had died.

I had received the message of his death as clearly as if it had been delivered by Western Union. I was puzzled, but I never questioned that unexplainable episode in my life.

A similar occurrence took place years later the day we buried my brother, Larry.

After his funeral I felt this strong urge to go to Larry's grave. I felt he was trying to tell me something, and the urge was so strong I dropped my wife and daughters off at my mother's and drove to the cemetery by myself.

It was late in the afternoon and the tent was still over the grave, the flowers surrounding it standing as an unbroken wall, and I knelt down beside the fresh grave.

"I'm here, Bud," I spoke quietly. "You wanted to tell me something?"

Of course I heard no words, but strong messages flowed into my mind. My brother was asking me to watch over his wife and family, to make sure they received their fair share from the business he had owned with partners. There were also a couple of personal messages, and when he was through my reporter training took over.

"Bud," I spoke the words aloud, "there's no question in my mind about the messages, but," I had to laugh, "if it's possible, could you give me a sign?"

On my left was this stand of flowers, outlined with fern. No sooner than I had finished the question, than a branch of the greenery snapped next to my left ear and fell to the ground.

I was shaken, stunned. I remained still for a short while and then I decided to repeat the question, to ask again for another sign, to be sure.

The afternoon was late, the air was still. Suddenly a

wave of wind washed across the grave, whistling with strength through the flowers, and it left as quickly as it came.

There was little doubt left in my mind of what had happened, but, as a reporter, I felt I must confirm, must be absolutely sure. Two or more sources, I grinned at the thought.

I stood up, walked around the grave, and stopped. "Bud," I said, "you know how stubborn I am. Could you give me one more sign?"

Near the fence bordering the cemetery was a pine tree. In this tree was a wild bluejay, squawking. The bird suddenly flew from the tree to the top of the fence post within two feet of me. Without fear, challenging me, this wild creature squawked and chirped loudly in my face. He was chewing me out, dressing me down, putting me in my place for doubting.

I turned back to the grave. "Even I can't deny this," I said. "Your message is loud and clear."

Satisfied, the bird flew away and I left the cemetery, my mind racing, trying to sort out what I had witnessed.

On the way home, on our trip back to Florida, I told the family what happened at my brother's grave, and daughters Karla and Alicia said later they didn't sleep very much during the rest of the trip.

The incident, like the overwhelming premonition that my son, Scott, had died, was kept within the family. It wasn't something to be shared with others. It was something that most likely would not have been believed in our circle of friends.

It is not my intention to try and convince you, to attempt to preach, or to influence your belief on the subject. It is only my intention to pass along to you all the things I utilized in my program to recover which may help you deal with coronary artery, or with any other disease. And faith in my opinion was an important component.

Now, when I go for walks, I gladly and sincerely give thanks to God for my health, for how He has blessed our family, for His will and the knowledge I have managed to gather to fight my inherited heart disease.

And as I go about my daily life I look for examples of God's intervention in healing, in answering prayers.

One touching incident I found out about concerns my
friend Kit Williamson, who is the former Deputy Police
Chief of our oceanside community, the city of Cocoa Beach.
During his life he has witnessed a great number of traffic
deaths. He has had the unpleasant and gut-wrenching duty
of pulling mangled bodies out of twisted and burnt metal.

Because of what he saw almost daily, he cautioned his
children, tried to make sure they drove defensely, gave themselves the best odds on the road.

His daughter Dorn heeded her father's advice, drove
sensibly, but no matter how careful a driver a person is,
there are accidents that are unavoidable.

Dorn Williamson was a senior at the University of Central Florida, and one Saturday evening she and friends were
returning from the beach on the two-lane State Road 520.
She was driving the speed limit, following a van.

The van, of course, blocked her view of on-coming traffic, but she kept her distance, kept in her lane, stayed with
the flow of traffic.

Suddenly, the van swerved to the right, off the road, and
Dorn and her friends stared at a pickup truck speeding head-
on toward them. There was no time to react. No time to
make a last-second attempt at avoidance.

The pickup truck slammed head first into Dorn's Monte
Carlo. Her seatbelt held her firmly, too firmly. Her head
snapped forward, whippedlashed backwards, then forward
again, then backwards, a repeated movement that swiftly
threw her into the black pit of unconsciousness.

Parts of her friends' bodies were crushed, bones broken,
flesh cut, but rescuers were able to pull them from the wreck
alive.

The driver of the pickup was killed instantly.

Dorn's fragile form was sandwiched between the seat
and the steering wheel and dashboard. It took rescuers three
hours to cut her free.

A rescue helicopter flew her to the main trauma center
in Orlando where she was hooked to tubes, sensors, and life
support machinery. She lay there, senseless, in a coma.

Her family stayed with her, stood watch by her bed.
There was no improvement.

The doctors told Kit she had contacted a septis infection. For thirteen days they searched for the source without success. All they could do was watch the infection destroy her vital organs.

Finally, the doctors called Kit and the family in and told them they had "maxed out." They had done everything they could do. Dorn was going to die.

Kit and the family were devastated with grief. They prayed and friends called for prayer services in local churches. There was a special mass at the local Catholic church, and in Georgia and Tennessee more churches were filled with prayer.

Friends in Europe lit candles in churches and Kit knelt by his daughter's bed. He had seen too much death. He knew what it looked like. It looked like Dorn.

He said his goodbyes, and went to the hospital chapel with his wife and son. They prayed.

The next morning, Dorn was still alive. The doctors were stunned.

The following morning she was still there, breathing but without any brain function. The brain waves were still flat.

They stayed by her bedside, and on the third day after the doctors had told them Dorn was going to die, her blood pressure returned to normal. The systolic had dropped to 40, dangerously low.

Her skin coloring was improving and a new doctor was brought in with a new drug. They tried it, and Dorn's infection was brought under control.

The family stayed with her. The prayers continued. More days passed and Dorn began to open her eyes. Suddenly, light made her blink. They all cheered.

The doctors told the family they weren't responsible. They had done everything they could, tried everything that medical science had to offer. "We didn't do it," they said. *"He did it."*

Dorn's brain function began to return and she was transferred to a rehabilitation center in Melbourne, Florida. Little by little she recovered, started talking, taking phone calls, and weeks later she returned to school where she was disappointed with a grade of B+.

She graduated with the loss of some of her vision and mobility, but today she lives a near normal life, and she's headed for graduate school.

Some will say Dorn would have recovered without prayer, but you won't convince the doctors attending her of that. Most medical professionals will tell you, they are not the last word. *He* is.

Another person you won't convince of that is former astronaut Jim Irwin whose walk on the moon I wrote about earlier. After my fall on the beach Jim and I got together to talk about his past experiences, his heart problems' and mine, and both of our near-death experiences.

Jim feels his life was saved by God in 1961. He had just graduated from test pilot school and considered himself one of the "hottest" pilots in the sky. One morning as he was flying with a student in a light aircraft, they crashed. The plane did not burn, but they were seriously injured—broken legs, broken jaws, many teeth gone, concussion, multiple lacerations. When Jim awoke in the hospital, doctors told him he probably would not fly again. You can imagine his despair.

Jim said he prayed and God made it possible for him to fly again, and his love for going fast and high led him to the space program.

It was ten years after the near-tragic accident that Jim Irwin went to the moon as lunar module pilot of Apollo-15; the longest of the lunar missions, the first to use a lunar car and the only one to visit the mountains of the moon—the journey when doctors first noted his heart problem.

Later, Jim experienced "sudden death," just as I did, while jogging. You will never convince him it was dumb luck that saved his life a third time.

As Jim and I talked about our experiences, the one major thing we agreed upon was that we both brought back from being clinically dead the total understanding that we were saved by God, that our experiences were in the hands of a higher authority.

What Jim remembers about his "sudden death" is only what he has been told by those who rescued him.

"I wish I could share all the events of that day with you, Jay," he told me, looking into my eyes, trying to focus on the past, "but I suffered a memory loss," he explained. "Three weeks wiped out. One week before, two weeks afterwards. Can't remember a thing."

What Jim was told by those who lived that day with him was that he had just returned from speaking at a luncheon, and, after putting on his jogging clothes, he started his run.

On the way down a dirt road from his home to the highway, he met his wife, Mary, who was returning from the grocery. They had house guests and he told her he would take everyone out to dinner after he returned from his jog.

Jim continued his run and when he reached the highway, he began his run up a hill, not a very steep hill, a hill he had run many times before.

This time, for some reason, his heart couldn't make it, and Jim collapsed, fell into the deep grass along the roadside, his legs sticking out on the highway.

Two young men came along, and moved his legs off the pavement and saw Jim wasn't breathing. They ran to a nearby house and called an ambulance.

The young men apparently didn't know what to do and this cost Jim Irwin precious time. He lay dead alongside the road for seven or eight minutes before the ambulance arrived and the emergency medical technicians began procedures to save him.

When they reached the hospital, Jim's heart was beating again, not very regularly, but it was beating.

His wife, Mary, had been called by the young men who spotted him. As soon as she got the word, she began praying. But Mary didn't stop with just her efforts. She notified prayer partners around the world and Jim Irwin's life was restored.

"Mary asked me if I had a life-after-death experience," Jim said. "Obviously I did, because when I became conscious I felt so calm," he added, "but I don't remember what it was."

There is much debate about what happens to people like Jim and me who are brought back from the dead—debate, generally, by people who are without experience.

I often see so-called experts on television talk shows explaining what takes place during "sudden death," and I find most of what they have to say amusing.

But when a person who has gone through such an experience is permitted to speak, there is suddenly a knowing, an understanding.

The one overriding common element from the experience is that each person returns not afraid of death. That's not to say we all want to go out and experience it all over again, because we all have things we want to do, loved ones we do not want to leave. But, when death comes, we know it's no big deal, and for us with *faith*—Christians, Jews, Buddhists, Moslems, all believers—even those who only possess an undefinable faith, we understand it is not the end. It's the entrance into another dimension, the beginning of another chapter in a person's existence.

Many feel faith, that is to say the strength of belief in your own mind, can make you well, or it can make you sick. They believe it is up to you. When your conscious mind programs your subconscious mind with the idea of good health, you will enjoy good health. But if you program your subconscious with fear and thoughts of disease, then you will most certainly become sick.

There is some scientific evidence to support this. Some people have pictured their diseases in their minds and have, during hours of meditation, visualized their diseases slowly disappearing.

Can picturing a cure help? I am unsure, but *faith* has been for me an important part in my program of self-managing my health, an important component of getting well.

SEVENTEEN

"Lookin' Good"

One year after falling on the beach, Jo prepared me the largest stack of pancakes I had ever seen. It was topped with bananas and a blueberry all-fruit spread, and, to my delight, one candle to celebrate the first birthday of my second life.

The family gathered around, took pictures, and we all laughed. It was a happy time. I had cheated death for another year, and my health was looking good. All was going well with my program, with my job, and I was passing "stress tests" like a Porsche passing other cars on a Florida highway.

Dr. Sarvanna Rajan was convinced our program of diet and exercise was reversing my coronary heart disease, and life was beautiful. It was time to live again, to be confident, to put disease and unpleasant thoughts behind us.

The passage of time was now convincing me that "sudden death" was a one-time experience, and my efforts to control my disease, and the encouraging results from those efforts, were further convincing me that I could now anticipate my future would be as guaranteed as most people's.

I looked up from my stack of pancakes at Jo. You could tell she too thought we again had a future, had more years together, and suddenly an idea that had been rolling around like a loose cannon in the back of my mind, leaped into words. "Let's get rid of this house."

She looked at me, face blanked, obviously caught by total surprise. "I thought you loved this house?"

"I do."

"You couldn't wait to live on the beach," Jo protested. "What about all the work we've put into it? What about that?"

"You've done a great job of decorating the Barbree Coast," I smiled, "but I'm ready for a more peaceful spot."

"The beach is peaceful."

"During the week," I argued. "Not on the weekend. It's all trashed by this spoiled society."

"I don't like picking up beer cans, bottles, food wrapers either," Jo said. "I just like this house."

"What about the traffic on A1A?"

"It's horrible."

"It's not gonna' get any better."

"No, I guess not," Jo agreed. "I just hadn't thought about it," she added, turning to study the house.

"Think about," I said. "Think about all the condos they're building, all that their gonna' build, and think about how there's no place to build new roads to handle all these people. There's only so much land."

"I know," Jo nodded. "It's terrible, and when all the " 'snow birds' " arrive, the beach is one huge parking lot."

I laughed. "That's why I make you do all the shopping."

"I've noticed that, but won't you miss all the traffic?" she laughed, knowing driving in traffic for me ranked right up there with a third-degree sunburn.

"Sure, like a rash I can't scratch."

"Well," she continued laughing, "I'll consider it as long as we can build our own place."

"Build?"

"Right! I want a California style home, and the only way we're gonna' get it around here is to build."

"I get my loft studio?"

"Uh huh," she smiled, her expression now one of serious but comfortable thought. "It could be like the house we've always wanted on a lake, big trees and all."

"Yeah, but there are no real lakes around here, no hills."

"I know," she said, "but we can still build the house."

"Right," I agreed, "We can still build the house."

Jo walked from the kitchen, to her desk in a small room she had set up as her own little office, and I knew she was already thinking, designing the house in her mind.

At the time, it seemed to me what we both needed were new goals, new projects, something that came with a future label on it. Something that helped us put uncertainty behind us. Put positive thoughts and plans ahead.

I also knew what I needed was a safe way to measure the growth, or lack of it, of the plaque within my coronary arteries. I could not let myself forget that the most important element of my health self-management plan was to make sure the lesions in my coronaries did not close. I had to be sure my diet and exercise program was working, but the only way to be positive was by risking another cardiac catheterization, the procedure that takes the life of one out of 2,000 who undergo it. I couldn't afford to *assume* everything was okay. I had to know. If I had a heart attack I might not get another chance.

I had been asking and looking for a non-invasive technique for months when one day the phone rang.

"Hello, Mr. Barbree?"

"Yes."

"My name is Tony Sintetos," the man said, "I understand from my uncle, Nick Pensiero, that you're looking for a way to keep check on your coronary lesions without catheterization?"

Nick Pensiero, the former head of Public Relations for RCA, had been my friend since the early days at the Cape and I was more than interested in what the man had to say.

"That's correct," I answered. "You say you're Nick's nephew?"

"Right," he assured me. "I'm with the Jacksonville Cardiovascular Clinic, and I may have something for you," he said. "I do angioplasty and caths up here."

"You a doctor?"

"Yes."

"But my doctor isn't planning a catheterization for me for another year."

"That may not be necessary."

"Really?" I was suddenly more than interested.

"You ever hear of a PETscan?"

"Yes, but just in passing," I told him.

"We're putting one in up here in conjunction with Jacksonville Memorial Hospital, and it should be ready in a few months."

"How is the PETscan different?"

"It can tell you the amount of blood flow you have through your coronaries without invading your body."

"It's safe?"

"Completely," he assured me.

I took a breath. "Sounds like something I should consider."

"Tell you what I will do," Dr. Sintetos said, "I will put your name on the list, and when we get the PETscan center open, we'll give you a call."

"Sounds great," I said, thanking him for calling, and putting the phone down with a new sense of relief.

Was this possible? Was there a non-invasive technique as reliable as the catheterization to keep track of coronary artery disease? Why hadn't I heard or read about this before? There was really no reason for me to doubt Dr. Anthony Sintetos. Hell, I'd known Nick Pensiero for thirty years. Nick knew as much about advanced technology as anyone.

I spent the next few days checking out the PETscan, learning all I could about the procedure and the opinions of many medical experts on the reliability of the new heart scanner.

What I learned was that doctors at Jacksonville's Memorial Medical Center were the third group, the third non-research hospital in the country, to buy one of the new $2.4 million PETscans, and I also learned some centers were fighting it because they had millions invested in less accurate equipment—investments they had to recover.

St. Joseph's in Atlanta and the renowned Cleveland Clinic in Ohio were the other two centers with the PETscan, but Jacksonville would be the first to offer heart scans on an outpatient basis.

Dr. David Hess, medical director of Jacksonville Memorial's Cardiac Catheterization Laboratory, said the PETscan center would be most interested in seeing patients who thought they might be at risk for heart disease, including those people with a family history of heart problems, high blood pressure or cholesterol.

Dr. Hess explained that PET was designed to detect heart disease in its earliest stages. It did it by generating color-coded, three-dimensional images that show a heart's structure, blood flow, and metabolism.

The scanner is basically a vertical, ring-shaped structure. A patient lies on a table that slides into the hole in the center of the ring so the chest is surrounded by the scanner.

The procedure on the device involves two scans in which a low-level radioactive tracer is injected into the bloodstream and remains in the body for four to six minutes. The scanner then watches the tracer as it moves through the heart, giving doctors a picture of the percentage of blood flow through the coronary arteries and any blockages that could lead to severe heart damage or heart attack.

The PET scanners have proved to be ninety-eight percent accurate, and are the most precise testing machines available to detect coronary artery disease in its earliest stages.

My doctors agreed I was a good candidate for the services of PET, and I was eager to take the test.

The call came for my appointment with the PETscan the last days of November 1988, the week of my fifty-fifth birthday.

The drive from the cape to Jacksonville was a routine trip northward along I-95, and when I reached the Jacksonville Memorial Medical Center, I was mildly surprised to find myself in what appeared to be a university complex, complete with a campus atmosphere.

The sprawling medical center occupies six blocks on the south side of the wide street, while doctors' offices, associated apartment complexes, and the Jacksonville Cardiovascular Clinic fill the north side.

I located the Memorial PETscan Center inside one of the huge buildings, and when I entered, I was immediately pleased with the decor. Nothing medical. Nothing hospital. Strictly a pleasant atmosphere staffed by pleasant people.

I signed in with Kay Hoover, the center's secretary and was quickly taken to a preparation room by Carol Foley, a pleasant RN who obviously flunked "nasty" when she went through nursing school. Her manner was more like that of an airline stewardess than that stereotyped "bossy nurse."

I was instantly and completely at ease. I really felt at home when Carol offered me a martial art's Gi to wear through the PETscan. She said the clothing was the most appropriate dress they could find for the test, and I quickly explained that since I had spent many years in the martial arts, I was very familiar with the Gi.

"With the what?" she asked.

"The Gi," I smiled. "That's what you call this garment."

"It is?" she laughed. "We didn't know what it was called," she confessed. "We were just pleased to find something that would suit our purposes."

"Whatever makes your boat float," I returned her laugh as she led me to a small room to change.

The dressing room offered the last moment to be alone with my thoughts and there was little question in my mind I had come to the right place. If the PETscan worked as advertised, I would soon know if my coronary disease had progressed, or if my efforts at diet, exercise, and good cholesterol numbers were paying off.

I left the dressing room eager to get started, and in only moments I was on a bed watching Carol take my vital signs.

When she was convinced I was alive, a hefty young man came into the room and positioned an xray camera over my chest.

"I have to locate the precise position of your heart, Mr. Barbree," he said. "This will help me position you just right in the PETscan."

"This is Mitch Lyle, Mr. Barbree," Carol explained. "He takes all the pictures and makes sure we do the test right."

"Hi, Mitch," I said. "Please call me Jay."

"Okay, Jay," the big man said. "We'll be ready for you as soon as Carol has done her thing."

Carol turned to me. "It's time," she said glumly, "for the only pain you will feel during the test."

"What's that?"

"I gotta' stick an I.V. in your arm," she said softly, her chin dropping to her neck.

"Oh, I think I can survive that," I smiled.

While she was busy searching for a good vein, a smartly dressed young man walked through the door followed by a smiling gentleman wearing a white smock. "Hi, Jay," the young man said, "I'm Patrick Thatcher, and this is Dr. Donald Gordon."

"Good morning," I greeted them, extending my right hand.

Patrick Thatcher is the center's public relations person and he had been most helpful in sending me a wealth of data and studies by independent universities on the PETscan. Dr. Gordon was the medical director of the PETscan center—the doctor who would be in charge of, and who would later review the results of, my exam—a warm and caring professional.

We were soon joined by cardiologist David Hess, a person I liked immediately, and both doctors began to run facts and figures on heart disease by me.

"The test with this nuclear scanner you are about to undergo, Mr. Barbree, can detect heart disease years before it can kill or disable its victims," Dr. Gordon told me, "and it does it without surgery."

"This is the first PETscan outpatient facility, right?" I asked.

"That's right," Dr. Hess joined in. "PET gives you color-coded, three-dimensional images of the heart—it's just like holding the heart in your hand," he explained. "It shows function, blood flow through the coronary arteries, and it shows metabolism of the heart muscle.

"PET can detect heart disease in its infancy, years before it might show up on a treadmill test, and years before it might cause chest pain or a heart attack."

"The PET scanner will have a profound impact on cardiology," Dr. Gordon predicted.

"It is a very important breakthrough in the diagnosis and evaluation of coronary heart disease," Dr. Hess added.

"I would much rather tell you that you have a fifty percent blockage in a coronary artery and closely watch that on a yearly basis, than to see you for the first time in the emergency room having a heart attack," Dr. Gordon said. "PET gives us the opportunity to treat the disease early in this silent stage, before you know it's there, with diet and exercise."

"You're getting no argument from me, doctors," I told them. "That's what I'm here for. I want to know what's there. What we have to deal with."

The two physicians looked at each other. "The trouble is only a small percentage of likely candidates for heart disease feel that way, Mr. Barbree," Dr. Hess said. "Most simply don't want to know. They deny they could have a problem until it's too late." He shook his head. "Forty percent of them don't make it through a heart attack."

Moments later, I was wheeled into the PETscan room where I was placed on a table that moved my head and shoulders through the large scan ring, leaving my heart encircled by the cameras.

Instantly I was aware how cold it was in the room. The temperature was kept low to make sure the cameras and computers worked efficiently, and Carol, the nurse Florence Nightingale must have had in mind, came to my rescue with heated blankets and a warm smile.

"Would you like to listen to some music during the test?" she asked.

"No, thank you," I said, rolling my head back and forth. "I'm comfortable."

"The cameras take a long time to take all the pictures we need," she explained.

"That's okay," I assured her, realizing that for some strange reason I was thinking I could help the process by concentrating.

I grinned at the idiotic thought, and Carol injected an radioisotope tracer through the I.V. into my arm. The safe dose of radiation is gone from the body within ten minutes, but as it moves through the heart, positrons (positively

charged electrons) are released. When a positron hits an ordinary electron, both are destroyed, giving off two gamma
rays which go in opposite directions. This provides a dual,
two-sided event to look at the coronary arteries. Only the
PETscan provides this full view of the heart.

Following the first scan, Carol injected a medicine
known as a "coronary vasodilator" into my arm. The medication has the same effect as an exercise stress test, but without
having to use a treadmill. It enlarges normal heart arteries,
increasing blood flow into the heart three to four times that
of treadmill or other stress tests.

The cameras were now taking a second PETscan of my
heart. If an artery is narrowed or blocked, the blood flow
will not increase as much to the area downstream of where
the narrowing or blockage is located.

Suddenly, I felt an unusual, and for me, strange pain,
"Dr. Gordon, there's a bizarre pain along my left side."

He was intently watching the monitors displaying my
heart's signatures. "How bad is it?" he asked.

"Not all that painful," I answered. "It's just a dull sort of
pain."

"Where do you feel it the most?"

"In my jaw," I said thoughtfully. "That's right, it's con-
centrated more in my jaw than anywhere else."

Dr. Gordon looked up at Carol. "We're two minutes into
the scan," he said, "go ahead and give him the antidote to the
Persantine."

"Don't worry, Jay," Carol smiled. "Two minutes is long
enough for us to get a good look at your heart." She smiled
again, placing her hand on my forehead. "This doesn't mean
you have a problem."

I looked up. "If he tells me I don't have a problem," I
grinned, "you'll see me jump through the ceiling."

Dr. Gordon smiled, knowingly, but Carol appeared puzzled. She was under the impression that I had walked in
from the street, a reporter who was interested in the PET-
scan, and curious as to whether he could have a problem.

I had not been totally honest with either of them. Dr.
Gordon knew I had dropped dead jogging, but he was not
aware of the advancement of my coronary artery disease. I

suppose he suspected I had a problem because of my bout with "sudden death," but he did not suspect I had six lesions growing on my arteries.

The exam was over. I changed back into my street clothes, and while I waited, Kay Hoover brought me a cup of coffee with some bran muffins. It was the first food for me of the day. My stomach was appreciative.

I finished the muffins, and enjoyed the last drop of the coffee before Dr. Gordon returned to lead me into a room where a TV monitor displayed color pictures of my heart.

Dr. Gordon explained what we were seeing, showed me precisely how life-giving blood flowed to my heart muscle. "Jay," he concluded, "you have coronary artery disease, but I'm not at all certain if it has progressed to the point where further action is necessary."

I was pleased with the PETscan results, and, for the first time, I brought out pictures of the catheterization by Dr. Narula following my "sudden death."

Dr. Gordon studied Dr. Narula's report, and I could tell by his expression he was puzzled. "The PETscan does not suggest," he said, "your coronary artery disease was anywhere as near critical as the catheterization has indicated."

I smiled at him. "What you are not aware of, Doctor," I told him, "is that I've been on a very low-fat diet for a year and a half, and I've lowered my cholesterol to around 150."

He looked up and nodded.

"I've also been able to raise my HDLs significantly, and with my brisk walking, Drs. Narula and Rajan feel we have at least halted the growth of my coronary disease."

"That's possible," Dr. Gordon said slowly. "I don't see your disease as severe today as your catheterization indicated."

"That's great," I told him. "It appears my efforts are paying off."

"I would say so," he smiled. "But I would like to study your exam further, have others take a look at it."

"The more input, the better," I agreed.

I left the PETscan center feeling great about the results, and follow-up letters from Dr. Gordon and Dr. Hess suggested I could safely stay on my diet and exercise program, and on the medication prescribed by Dr. Narula, for another year before I should undergo another PETscan.

A year may not seem long to most people, but when you are living with a life-threatening disease, it's a lifetime.

When I got home, Jo wasn't there, and I didn't bother going inside. Instead, I went for a quiet walk on the beach. I had this overwhelming urge to be alone, to reflect on all that I had seen and experienced that day. I was thankful to God for a machine such as the PETscan. I could readily see how it could safely keep track of my disease without having to undergo the risky catheterization. I had the feeling it was going to play a big role in my future. At the moment, I had no idea how big.

I stopped at the crossover, again admiring the coconut palms I had planted. Like me, they appeared healthy, growing and spreading their long fronds.

"You guys," I smiled down at them, "will go with me to the new house."

EIGHTEEN

"Return to Flight"

Astronaut Michael Coats kept his vision moving across the controls to the array of gauges on the instrument panel before him. He didn't study the gauges. You didn't do that because when you were flying the space shuttle, the most sophisticated high-tech machine ever created, you surveyed what was before you. Concentrate on one instrument, and you ignored the others. So you kept up a scan; your practiced eye picked out things that were wrong and paid scant or no attention to what was right.

It was no easy task at the moment. On our way into orbit we had lost two main engines. They had shut themselves down prematurely, and we no longer had the energy to reach space. We had to turn around and we were returning to the launch site, lining up with the Kennedy Space Center's shuttle landing strip.

The procedure is called an RTLS—Return to Launch Site Abort, and Mike Coats was in the commander's seat. I was seated in the pilot's chair, and I was admiring every move of the skilled test pilot. His fingers were those of a master musician, deft and dexterous, knowing that the slightest movement on the shuttle's controls could change the shuttle's delicate, computerized approach.

"Discovery, your energy is good, you're on glidescope."

"Roger, Houston."

The runway was dead ahead and my feet were on the

rudders, following Astronaut Coats' every move. I had taught instrument flying on simulators in the Air Force, but this shuttle job was too real. If it had not been for Dave McCollum, the producer, and cameraman Hal Leibowitz and crew looking over my shoulders, it would have been easy to imagine I was actually in the pilot's seat of a space shuttle.

But I wasn't. It was a shuttle simulator, and NBC News and other major news organizations had been invited to take a simulator ride with an astronaut.

Lucky me. I had drawn the assignment and as I glanced over my shoulder at my good buddy Dave McCollum, I saw a face filled with envy. He wanted to be in that seat. He too was a pilot, a former C-131 driver who spent several years in the Air Force pushing the big cargo jets across the sky.

I thought about exchanging places with Dave, but it was too much of a technical hassle, and he understood. He wasn't happy, but Dave understood.

Mike Coats landed the shuttle simulator dead center of the runway, and our ride was over . . . too quickly over.

We all took a deep breath and Hal rolled tape and I began the interview. Questions about how the astronauts trained on the simulator, and questions about any lingering doubts following the Challenger accident that Mike Coats, or any of the astronauts, may have regarding the risks of flying the space shuttle.

Afterwards, I had a few moments to talk with Mike Coats, to thank him for the ride, and to wish him well on his upcoming shuttle flight.

He knew I was a finalist in the Journalist-in-Space Project, and because I had been a pilot, he wished me luck. He said he would be happy to have me as a member of his crew anytime, and I appreciated the kind gesture even though it may have only been a well-mannered passing offer.

I was very aware most astronauts are against flying civilians on the shuttle, and I was also very aware the likelihood I would ever get that opportunity were slim. NASA wasn't likely to permit a reporter with coronary artery disease to fly in space, and I was beginning to regard my chances of reaching orbit as an once-in-your-life-adventure that could have been.

But David Garrett at NASA Headquarters in Washington, assured me the Journalist-In-Space project was still very much alive even though it was on hold, and, after the Teacher-In-Space flew, a journalist would head into orbit.

In regard to my medical condition, Garrett said I was still a finalist, and the issue of my medical predicament would be settled by the Aerospace Medicine Board.

Billie Deason of the Public Affairs Office at the Johnson Space Center in Houston told me that the Aerospace Medicine Board must review and pass on every person who goes into space. "The doctors here tell me that a person who has had a cardiac arrest as you did," she added, hesitantly, "that would be a negative, not a plus."

It was just a nice way of telling me I was still in the project, but I was hanging on with the weakest of grips.

Despite my good intentions to be more mellow, I found myself covering the space shuttle flights with the same tenacity and urgency I had before. I was, without question, reverting back to many of "the old ways." Stress and hostile reactions to things not going right were again part of my life, and I found myself violating my diet not just occasionally but frequently.

Between shuttle missions I was able to keep pretty much to my diet and exercise program, but during the launches, when I was at Press Site #39, where NBC had our food catered, I found myself at the feeding trough all too often.

The food was tempting. High fat meals prepared to please the customer, strictly no regard for health.

Sometimes I complained about what we were being fed. In fact, I named the caterer "Cholesterol Mary," but I was told to keep quiet—told by my supervisors I might hurt her feelings.

I grunted to myself. That's what I was trying to do in a twisted sort of way. I was trying to get the message across that fat is a poison, that it kills. I was outvoted, and the animal flesh smothered in melted cheeses and swimming in fat kept coming and I kept eating perhaps to compensate or indulge or as a matter of convenience, and a lack of discipline.

Going into space had been a magnificent dream, but NBC News wasn't paying me to dream. I was being paid to cover the space program, to keep up with every minute detail of the resumption of space shuttle missions. And I tried to refocus my attention on that job.

NASA officials had been shaken by the Challenger accident, and Rear Admiral Richard Truly, an experienced shuttle pilot, was named to direct the shuttle program; several other astronauts were placed in key management positions. There were wholesale resignations and shifting of duties at the Marshall Space Flight Center and Morton Thiokol, the overseers and builders of the shuttle booster rocket that failed.

The directors of the Marshall, Kennedy and Johnson centers all left, and later, Admiral Richard Truly became the top boss, the Administrator of NASA.

To correct the rocket joint problem, engineers added a third O-ring seal, a metal capture lip to prevent joint rotation at ignition, improved insulation, heaters to warm the joints in cold weather like the freezing temperatures that had affected Challenger, and a dozen other changes. They also made improvements to the shuttle's main engines, brakes and landing gear, and they added an explosive-charged blowout hatch to the cabin. The hatch would not help in a Challenger-like situation, and would be for use only during an emergency landing incident when a shuttle was gliding toward a touchdown and the astronauts could bail out.

In all, the three remaining shuttles underwent a $2.4 billion overhaul, with a total of fifty-six major design changes.

Following the January 28, 1986 Challenger accident, NASA said it might be able to resume flights as early as July 1986. But as the magnitude of the overhaul became apparent and as more failed tests occurred schedules slipped; the projected launch date was delayed to February 1988, then to June, to July, to August, and finally September.

But like me, the program finally was reborn. On the morning of September 29th, 1988, the space shuttle Discovery sat on its launch pad, its huge external fuel tank overflowing with 500,000 gallons of liquid hydrogen and liquid oxygen fuels, its crew cabin inhabited by five seasoned shuttle astronauts.

The crew was commanded by Navy Captain Frederick H. "Rick" Hauck.

With Hauck were Air Force Colonel Richard O. Covey, the pilot, and mission specialists George D. "Pinky" Nelson, John M. "Mike" Lounge and Marine Lt. Colonel David C. Hilmers.

More than a million people lined riverbanks, roadways, and causeways. More than 2,400 news media representatives from around the world were on hand to record and report NASA's comeback. Excitement, tempered by the memories of *Challenger,* rose as the countdown entered the final hours.

The weather around Launch Pad 39B was excellent. But 20,000 to 50,000 feet overhead, it was not all right. The winds, surprisingly, were too tame for the time of year, spring-like instead of fall-like. Discovery's computers had been programmed to maneuver the craft through strong, buffeting winds. It would take at least a day to reprogram them. The countdown was held while weather balloons were sent up to monitor the winds.

Inside Discovery's cabin, Commander Rick Hauck looked at his crew. "We're not going anywhere today, guys," he said.

The crew listened while launch director Robert Sieck tried to come up with a solution, tried to save the day.

Again the crew smiled. "No way," said Pilot Dick Covey.

"Crip wont let us fly in this weather," Commander Hauck assured the rest.

Crip, veteran shuttle astronaut Robert Crippen, was wearing the hat of deputy operations manager and was charged under new management rules with giving the final go-no-go for launch.

The crew waited in silence, waited for a report back from the weather balloons, when suddenly, pilot Dick Covey who was looking out the window, said "Uh oh!"

"Uh oh, what?" Rick Hauck's question was immediate and tense.

"I see a cloud over there," Covey said. "Could be problems."

"Dick," Commander Hauck shouted. "You don't say " 'Uh oh' " on top of a rocket filled with a half a million gallons of fuel."

They all laughed, and the sudden tension was broken. "Don't worry about it guys," Covey said. "Crip's not gonna' let us go anywhere today."

"Yeah, we'll be outta' here in a few minutes," Hauck again assured them.

Before long, the winds did shift and pick up a little, but they were still outside NASA's criteria for liftoff. After a detailed analysis, the mission management team determined the shuttle had sufficient structural margin and was not endangered. Astronaut Robert Crippen surprised the launch team, surprised us long-time observers at the press site, and most of all surprised the crew. He gave the final *"go"* for launch.

The astronauts looked at each other, swallowed hard, and Commander Rick Hauck said, "Let's go flying, guys."

Inside the NBC News complex, we were overrun with executive types from the network, and a variety of correspondents had been sent out to cover every element of the story. My job was to keep up with the story, to stay on top of every decision launch managers were making, and once the flight was underway, I was to handle the live, extended radio program.

I had been given the studio for the major program and three other radio correspondents set up outside to do their individual reports. Everything was in place and I was trying to monitor what was happening in launch control, keep in touch with my sources, trying to stay on top of the story.

"Jay, I'll bet this is old hat to you by now?" one of the editors asked.

"Not really," I smiled. "I never tire of watching the launches," I answered, leaning my ear closer to the launch control speaker, trying to hear Hugh Harris' running commentary.

"Jay," someone else said, "Now don't forget you have a cutaway after the solid boosters burn out."

"Right."

"How far is it to the launch pad, Jay?"

"About four miles."

"What was the most exciting launch you ever covered?"

"This one ranks up there," I said, still trying to smile. "Please, let me monitor launch control. We've gotta' keep up with the story."

"Lou wants a spot right after the launch, Jay."

"Okay."

"You think it will go today?"

"I think so now that we've gone passed T-minus 9 minutes," I said, pleading once again to be permitted to listen.

I knew the visiting editors and producers were good people, they were just interested in every little fact, use to working in a big city news room where people are never considerate. The more noise the better. Well, that wasn't how it was with me. I worked alone, and when I was set upon by all these meaningless questions, not permitted to concentrate on the story, I began to climb the walls.

I was known as the correspondent who threw a Chicago editor out of the trailer during the Gordon Cooper Mercury flight, and my tolerance level was peaking. It was time to throw a whole bus load out.

"*OUT,*" I screamed, the single word bouncing off the walls and studio window with enough force to spread the sound across the press mound. "How in the hell do you expect me to keep up with what's going on if I've gotta' answer every dumb question passing through your minds?"

The radio people were shocked, including my wife who had been brought out to keep us in groceries and drink. They weren't too sure if I was serious or not. "To answer you peoples' next dumb question, no I do not know who was the first person to *fart* in space. I suspect it was Yuri Gargarin who was the first one up there, but I'm only guessing, okay?"

They all stared at me, wondering if there was something to be said.

I managed a smile, lowered my voice. "Please," I said. "I ask you one more time, please let me think. Let me listen to launch control. Let me keep up with the story. The launch could have been scrubbed and we wouldn't know it!"

The room cleared, and I picked up Hugh's commentary, settled into my chair before my microphone. Moments later I received my cue and I went on the air, bridging between what Hugh Harris was telling us and what I witnessed from my vantage point.

At 11:37 A.M., ninety-eight minutes late, Discovery's main engines and rocket boosters roared to life and the huge space plane rose majestically from a pillow of fire and steam. Hugh Harris' voice quivered as he choked out the words, "Liftoff, we have liftoff. Americans return to space as Discovery clears the tower."

The assemblage of more than one million—one out of every two hundred fifty Americans—crossed their fingers, gritted their teeth, clenched their fists, as they watched the shuttle thunder ever higher on its seven hundred-foot pillar of fire.

I too crossed my fingers as I shouted words into my microphone, attempting to paint a verbal picture for our audience as every second the booster rockets burn seemed to grow longer and longer. When Discovery reached the plus 73 second point, the spot in the sky where the Challenger Seven died, Rick Hauck acknowledged mission control's transmission with the same words spoken at the same point in Challenger's flight by commander Dick Scobee: "Roger, go at throttle up," Hauck said with remembrance and respect.

For our audience, I kept counting off each second the astronauts had remaining on their ride with the boosters, and when the rockets, blamed for the *Challenger* accident, burned out as scheduled and peeled away, there were cheers all across the press site.

Six and one-half minutes later, the main engines shut down and Discovery settled into an orbit one hundred eighty miles high. Again cheers erupted from the press site, and from the launch control and mission control centers.

I wrapped up the program, signed off, and slumped back into my chair. NASA was back in space, and I was back covering the shuttle flights with the same tenacity and urgency I had before. I was, without question, reverting back to many of "the old ways." Stress and hostile reactions to things not going right were again part of my life.

As the weeks passed, the shuttles kept flying and the awareness of my coronary artery disease grew dimmer in my mind. The good PETscan report had given me confidence that I had arrested the growth of the disease, and as long as I kept passing my treadmill stress tests and my cholesterol numbers stayed in check, I felt confident.

Jo and I sold our home on the ocean, and, after spending weeks looking for the right spot to build our new home, we heard of Honeymoon Lake on south Merritt Island.

"Take a drive on Stillwaters Drive," friends told us. "You'll like it."

To get there, we drove along South Tropical Trail, a winding roadway covered with trees and tropical greenery on the banks of the Banana River. It wasn't a road to hurry along, but a road without bumper-to-bumper traffic; an isolated road that seemed far removed from the hustle and bustle of the tourist dollar; reaching back through the decades to a time the heart wasn't called on to beat very fast.

When we reached Hilltop Drive and drove onto the street, we both were very pleased to find hills, what some folks in the area call Merritt Island's mountains; not hills as thought of by most in other parts of the country, but hills nevertheless—hills rising above Florida's normal flat terrain.

We drove through the entrance of Stillwaters Drive and found ourselves on a beautiful winding street that flowed downward through large oaks to the lake, by homes well kept on acre lots situated along the shore.

Jo looked at me. "This is beautiful," she said, "I never knew there was a place like this in the area."

"I didn't either," I said quietly, searching each side of the private drive for a vacant lot.

Folklore says Honeymoon Lake, a mile long and about half that wide, was carved out by a meteor crashing to earth millions of years ago. The meteor cut the lake alongside the Indian River and pushed the land there to the east, creating rolling hills reaching to the island's other side where it meets the Banana River.

A NASA engineer was holding onto the lot next to him, and we convinced him to sell.

Jo and I were happy. We had located a place to build where God's creations grew, not where the only growth was concrete and condos.

The days continued to pass and we were busy designing and building our dream house—a house with rooms and space we had always envisioned, but were never able to find.

Frequently we found ourselves disagreeing over the "small stuff," over details that really meant very little, but, out of respect for Jo's ability to decorate and my need to live stressfree, I decided the details would be left to her judgement.

The only real conflict that arose was, of all things, over the coconut palms. Jo insisted that they would not go with our landscaping on the lake, and, of course, I disagreed.

"There are all sorts of tropical plants along Tropical Trail," I argued, "including coconut trees."

"They will look ridiculous with the oaks," Jo said, irritated with my insistence. "Leave them where they are."

I left one coconut palm for the Sileos, but, as I had promised the trees, I brought three with me to the island.

I tried to stay out of Jo's, and friend Henry Goolsby's, way when it came to the new house, but I did beg for the right to have a say in my own studio, my hideaway loft to write, the place to broadcast many of my radio reports.

I think I won that right! I'm not sure. It could be Jo was just letting me think I did.

I knew our friend Henry Goolsby was a solid builder and I

kept my distance, watched the construction, and found I really had nothing to complain about. Henry and Jo were doing great. It was a delight to watch the new home rise.

What I wasn't pleased with was my backsliding to old habits of diet, and actions like reacting hostilely to pressure, to traffic, and to company politics.

The shuttle flights were taking place almost as often as they had before the Challenger accident, and the long hours needed to keep in front of the competition were again part of my life.

When it came to space coverage, I was keeping NBC out front, but every time I came up with a real, solid exclusive the producers in New York would ask me to pass it along to another correspondent.

The "big footing," the plagiarism of the fruits of my journalistic skills, was tearing my heart out. Something had to change if I was to ever again have peace of mind.

I had accumulated three weeks of vacation time and the company began to insist I take it, otherwise I was going to lose it.

Son Steve in Illinois and our wonderful daughter-in-law, Norma, had given us a new grandson, Brian, and we were most anxious to see him as well as granddaughters Bethney and Michelle.

We met them in a wonderful place in the smokies named "Deer Ridge," where we spent a most enjoyable week.

Steve, far more level-headed and laid back than his dad, talked with me about the "big footing" problem with the company.

We walked through the mountains, along isolated and peaceful trails, and Steve helped me to understand that life wasn't fair, that the world is overrun with insensitive people. He pointed out the best I could hope for was to continue to do my best as a reporter, to serve NBC News in any capacity the company had in mind.

"They have to compete in an unforgiving arena, dad," Steve said. "They need to take their best shot, and if that best shot means feeding your exclusive information through another mouth, then you've gotta' be part of the team."

"You're right, son," I said. "But we all grew up within the business with certain ethics, with professional principles that meant something." I stopped in the middle of the trail. "There was nothing in the rules that said a reporter could only be

young, could only be pretty, could only speak through a mouthful of capped teeth."

"Age and wisdom has its place," Steve smiled, "but the producers in New York have their own set of unique problems. Show
business plays a role, dad, that you've gotta' understand."

"I do, son," I said. "The business is changing, nothing stays
the same."

"And you must change with it," he patted me on the back.
"You must realize there are some mountains that can't be
climbed. There are some things that just can't be changed."

"And I should have the wisdom to know the difference," I
interrupted thoughtfully.

I doubt if Steve knew how much he helped me that week in
the Smokies, but I had a fresh attitude, the importance of which
was becoming more clear to me. I was simply going to do my
best, be a team player, and help the company be a news leader
in every way I could. But even while I had been adopting Steve's
advice as to attitude, my acquired habit of healthful food continued to slip.

A few months before I had discovered no-fat frozen yogurt,
and almost every day of the three-week vacation, I pigged out on
the frozen delight. Under the guidelines of my diet, I could see
no wrong in eating it, but, because of it and other diet violations,
I was regaining weight.

I was disappointed in myself for my lack of discipline, but
surprised the medication was still keeping my cholesterol numbers in a good range.

It was time to return to work, but more importantly, it was
time to get back on my rigid diet, to get ready for my second
PETscan. I wanted to give the second exam every chance to be
as good as the first.

I felt somewhat guilty I had not been as faithful to my diet
as I had been the first year and a half after I collapsed on the
beach, but I was still confident my coronary disease was in
check. Perhaps it had not reversed itself, but I had faith it would
be no worse.

NINETEEN

"The Setback"

The cameras within the giant PETscan ring hummed in a constant voice as they scanned my flesh and blood, sinew and tendon and muscle, veins and arteries and nerves, bone and marrow, pulsing liquid flow, the trillions of cells that are my body, and fed the information to the computer. The computer digested what it saw, and reduced the information to only the pictures of the heart, of the blood flow through the organ, and recorded it on video tape for later study by Dr. Donald Gordon.

My mind flowed with the noise of the PETscan, confident it would be the first of many routine tests that would prove my coronary artery disease was in check.

By this time, more than two years had passed since my sudden death on the beach, I definitely thought of that close call as an isolated event. My latest stress tests, both on treadmill and the nuclear reading on a stationary bicycle, had conveyed to Dr. Saravanna Rajan that my disease was under control. In fact, the nuclear stress exam just two months before had shown no sign of heart disease.

"If I didn't know it was you," Dr. Ragan had told me, "I would send this person home with the knowledge he was completely free of heart disease."

"It's that good?" I asked.

"It's that good," he said. "No sign of any disease at all," he smiled. "I think the lesions are in regression."

I could not have been more pleased. I was convinced my research, and the knowledge developed by university and medical centers, had given me the program needed to control coronary artery disease.

Even my cholesterol that morning had reported in at an all time low—138. The technicians in the lab were so astonished they ran the blood sample through the lab again, just to be sure.

Everyone was smiling, especially Jo. She had come along to Jacksonville with me just to see the PETscan Center, to get a look at the Jacksonville Cardiovascular Center I had been bragging about.

And for some reason, this second time, the PETscan room didn't seem so cold, but nurse Carol Foley was there, making sure all was running smoothly.

It was. That is it was until we entered the second phase of the scan, until Carol dumped the vasodilator (Persantine) into my I.V. . Only seconds passed before an unusual feeling rushed through my stomach, a sort of empty, nauseated feeling that seem to want to send up whatever I had in my stomach, but, thankfully there was nothing there. Instead the feeling produced a dull pain that began to spread up my body, through my arms, and into my jaws.

The vasodilator medication had increased the blood flow to my heart by three to four times. The result was to simulate exercise I could never achieve on a treadmill. My legs would give out first, but this time, on the PETscan, I knew Dr. Donald Gordon was watching a true picture of my coronary artery disease.

"That pain is back," I told him.

He glanced up from the monitor. "Same as before?"

"About the same."

"Where do you feel it most?"

"In my left side, my left arm, but mostly in my jaws," I said.

"You want to stop the test?"

"No," I told him. "I want to finish this time."

"Didn't we finish the first one?"

"No," I assured him. "You ordered Carol to administer the antidote about two minutes in."

"Not according to this," he said, nodding at his chart. "According to this we finished."

"We completed the first test," Carol agreed.

"No," I disagreed. "We stopped after two minutes and you told me that was enough to get the results."

They both looked hazy. I felt the issue wasn't worth pursuing and I let it drop. It was clear in my mind that we had not completed the four-minute period with the vasodilator, and this time, if the pain permitted, I wanted to finish. I felt that as long as Dr. Gordon was reading my real time EKG, we would be okay.

I kept squeezing the hand grip and the pain settled into a constant level, my jaws feeling like I had just chewed two packs of chewing gum without a break. It wasn't something I could not stand, but for me it was unusual. I was a victim of silent ischemia and I had never experienced angina.

Soon, the four minutes had passed and Carol administered the antidote through the I.V. and I waited for it to reverse the pain. It didn't. I looked at her and Dr. Gordon. "The pain is still there," I said. "It's not going away as it did before."

Dr. Gordon appeared puzzled. "Give him another dose," he ordered.

Carol sent the antidote rushing through the I.V. tube and seconds later the dull pain was swept from my body. The blood flow through my arteries was normal, and I felt like my old self. It was time to leave the PETscan table and wait for the results.

Jo and I sat in the conference room drinking our coffee and enjoying one of those delicious bran muffins as we waited for the results of the PETscan. I wasn't the least bit concerned about the dull pain I had felt during the second phase of the exam. I had felt it before with good results, and with the results of my treadmill stress tests, there appeared to be no cause to worry.

Then the minutes grew into hours. Apprehensive, I got up and went out into the hall. I hailed Dr. Gordon who was walking by. "What does it look like?" I asked.

He didn't answer immediately. He stared straight ahead. "I don't give preliminary reports," he said. "I'll have everything ready in a few minutes."

I watched as he walked through the door into the room where the PETscan's monitors were located. A feeling I didn't care for swept through my body. That feeling of being *alone* again. Suddenly and painfully I felt something was wrong. I could only hope it wasn't too serious. I could only hope I had not lost ground during the past year. I could only hope my condition was still manageable.

I walked back in the conference room and sat down. Jo and Carol were busy with conversation and I really didn't want to alarm them. But, as I listened to Carol, I could detect concern in her voice. She had been in the monitor room, possibly had seen the results, but she couldn't say anything until Dr. Gordon was ready.

Finally Dr. Gordon came to the door and signaled Jo and me to follow him into the monitor room.

As we entered, I could see the animation that was my heart on the screen. I studied it. I could not see anything wrong. I felt better.

Dr. Gordon placed us in chairs on each side of him and he began explaining what we were seeing on the monitor. Everything appeared normal during the first phase of the exam "Jay" he said quietly "your heart seemed to be getting a normal supply of blood. It was only when during the second phase of the test, if you look at the blood flow, that the results became obvious. Blood flow to the bottom half of your heart" he pointed meaningfully "totally and completely disappeared. At peak exercise, forty-six percent of your heart was being denied blood, an indication that the upper two lesions were closing up."

He didn't have to say anything more.

I spoke for him. "There's no blood reaching the lower

part of my heart at this level of exertion," I said quietly. "That's a major change. That's a major problem."

"That's right," he confirmed.

Numbness replaced all feeling in my body. My mind shifted into a defensive mode. Here I was all *alone* again. Here I was faced with the horrible reality that *death* was once again an unwelcome visitor about to knock on my door.

What had been an upbeat future for the last year—a future that included a new house to go along with what I felt was new-found health and a good job—had instantly vanished as if it had only been a wisp of midnight fog that had temporarily settled before being blown away by an ocean breeze.

I glanced quickly at Jo. She sat there puzzled, but aware of what we were seeing. She knew my life was being threatened again, and it would, most likely, take strong measures to overcome this new, yet old threat.

I turned to Dr. Gordon, "What do we do?"

"You need another cathetcrization," he said flatly but firmly "You need to know how much those upper lesions have progressed."

There seemed little doubt in his mind, and there was really little that wasn't apparent to me. What I had feared for years was suddenly a reality. I was on the verge of a major, life-threatening heart attack and I did not like the feeling that had invaded my mind, drained my energy, and left me feeling frightened and alone.

I looked around me. The faces were suddenly no longer the same friendly, out-going and social ones I had seen there earlier that morning. Instead there were eyes filled with pity, there were voices that made every attempt to say just the right thing, there were human beings who were thankful those pictures were not of their heart.

In spite of the numbness that swept my body I suddenly felt uncomfortable around people, unable to really carry on a sincere conversation. I truly felt unwelcome, sensed a sort of group feeling that they all preferred I would go away. I was suddenly the cripple in a wheelchair, the disabled on crutches, the reminder that we are all fragile, not one of us is perfect, and I was a threat to each person's belief in their own perfection.

But I did not have time to concern myself with the pity of others, with that sense I was a dead rat being carried outside between the firm fingers of someone holding their nose. It was time for me to think, to cut through the devastating numbness, and to deal with my predicament.

What had always been one of my strengths was to seek a way up in spite of the hill to be climbed, and I suddenly remembered a definition of life I had always admired. "Survival is the simple art of getting up just one more time than you have been knocked down."

I encouraged myself. Get up, Jay, and find the answers.

I rose from my chair. "Would you call Dr. Hess and see when he will be available to perform a catheterization on me?" I asked Dr. Gordon.

He attempted a smile. "Certainly," he answered. "That should be your first step."

"Salvage what is salvageable," I nodded.

"That's right," Dr. Gordon assured me. "I'll have Dr. Hess take a look at your PETscan and we'll take it from there."

A couple of hours later Jo and I were on our way home, driving down I-95. We said little. We both were considering the chores we had to get done before the catheterization. I had to take the time off from work, we had to tell the family, and we had to clear our appointments for work on the house as well as prepare for what would follow the catheterization —the procedure that would be necessary to restore blood flow to my heart.

Would angioplasty do the job? Would open heart surgery be necessary? Before I permitted my thoughts to travel along those paths too far, I reminded myself that I should call Dr. Narula as soon as I got home.

What would he think? All our stress tests had been successful. I was able to walk briskly for more than three miles without the slightest fatigue. I was a picture of health. In fact I hadn't felt so good in many years.

What the hell, I thought. Could the PETscan be wrong? I knew the answer to that. The chances were one in a hundred, and I also knew of many examples where a person had passed a treadmill stress test only to drop dead with a heart attack hours or days later.

As we have written Jim Fixx, expert and author on jogging, fell dead while running. Joe Morrison, head football coach at the University of South Carolina, collapsed in a shower and died of a heart attack after playing racquetball. Basketball star "Pistol" Pete Maravich died playing basketball, pop singer Roy Orbison, Chicago Mayor Harold Washington, Baseball Commissioner Bart Giamatti, the list goes on. All of these victims were in their fifties and routinely had access to physicals.

If the catheterization scheduled with Dr. Hess in two days confirmed the PETscan, then it would be clear that all the treadmill tests had been useless.

"Under the best, optimum conditions a treadmill stress test is only about fifty percent accurate," Dr. Hess told me. "That means fifty patients out of a hundred with heart disease who had a treadmill test are walking around with severe heart disease thinking they are okay," Dr. Hess explained. "I have seen hundreds of patients in the emergency room suffering a heart attack who had a negative treadmill test a few days before."

I shuddered at the thought. If I had accepted the results of my stress tests as gospel, I would now be living my last weeks, certainly months of life. And, of course, if something could not be done to restore blood flow to my heart, then . . .

Our drive home continued. We both were locked in silent thought. It was difficult for Jo and me to talk after our feelings had been so numbed by reality. We both were so convinced all our efforts had my coronary disease under control. Jo had been such a helpful partner. Preparing my low-fat meals, making sure I had time for my walks, helping me follow my program religiously.

The one question that kept running through my mind,

the same question that I refused to think about, was: Was it possible my program had failed me altogether? Was it possible all of the dieting, the lowering of my bad cholesterol, the raising of my good cholesterol, the exercise, the lowering of my weight, had had little effect on my coronary artery disease?

The farther I drove the more the confused thoughts ran together, the more unclear they became. I found myself simply wanting to get home, to reach my bed, to be *alone* with my aloneness. Perhaps sleep would wash away the numbness. Perhaps not. There was so much to think about. Many decisions to be made. I drove and permitted myself to steal a line from Scarlet O'Hara. "I'll think about *that* tomorrow."

TWENTY

"Why"

Tomorrow came and I still didn't want to think about it! For most of the past two-and-a-half-years despite my recent dietary lapses I had been following the best plans researchers and medical science had to offer to control coronary artery disease, and the God-awful truth was that it hadn't worked.

Even though my weight was creeping up, I had lowered my cholesterol to an unbelievable 138, replaced up to half of it with the healthy HDL cholesterol, kept my blood pressure normal—sometimes below normal—exercised properly, and attacked fat as if it was poison. So, what went wrong?

If the PETscan was right, then it would appear all these herculean efforts were wasted. It appeared no matter what I had done or what I would do would make any difference. It was as if my body had been programmed to produce coronary artery disease that would take my life in my fifties. After all, that's what had happened to my father, to his brothers, to my own brother, and to two of my cousins.

Was I really just kidding myself with all these precautions? Had I been denying myself for no real reason? Was I being a fool to think one could overcome heredity?

I didn't really want to think about this, I really didn't want to believe that I had been wrong, that all my efforts had been wasted.

But I didn't have a choice. I had to think about it. I had

to try and make sense of what was happening to me, of the disease that was eating its way through my coronary arteries.

As was my habit, I had chosen a walk on the beach to clear my mind, to digest the facts.

There was something about the warm sun, the sand beneath my feet, the crashing of the surf that helped me think. I suppose it was the complete environment; the squeals of the seagulls over my head, the laughter of children near and far, distant sounds of airplanes and automobiles, and a faint drift of music. Closer sounds, the sea breeze whipping past my body, the soft slap of my feet on wet sand. What a marvelous, wonderful life.

Could what the PETscan revealed be signalling the end of it?

Among the questions and the sounds of children laughing it seemed as if I could hear the words of my own father. Saying, "I told you so."

He had been a "hardshell" Baptist and they believe "What will be, will be." He was convinced that there was one big plan that affected each individual, and, no matter what you did, there was no way you could change it.

My father believed that the day you were born, the time and method you would die had already been predetermined. He believed that while you were on this earth, your main purpose should be to live a "good" life, and to please God to the best of your ability.

I had to grin. Could he have been right?

I didn't believe it, I answered my own question quickly. It is difficult not to believe that man has his own fate in his hands. He has the choice to do good, or to do evil. He has the choice to use the brain God gave him to improve his life, to help others, to advance medical knowledge, to save and extend life.

I stopped my walk for a moment, turned and faced the ocean. It would have been easy for me to unleash my disappointment, to let self-pity and hostility drench my body. It would have even felt good to kick a door in—to break a chair over something, to take my frustrations out on something that couldn't fight back.

I shook my head and turned back to resume my walk. I searched my inner feelings only to find my mood was one of puzzlement, of questioning, of seeking new answers. Not one of anger.

I had been convinced that I had found the answers in my research over the past two-and-a-half-years, and possibly I had. Just because the program to fight heart disease that I had so carefully worked out with Dr. Narula and others hadn't worked for me, didn't mean it was a failure. What I had to remember was that the data only promised it was a protection for two out of three people, and suddenly it was clear that I was the one out of three it didn't help. Or did it?

I stopped my walk again. Stood solidly on the sand. How was I to know that if I had not followed my diet, had not lowered my cholesterol, exercised, kept a healthy blood pressure, that I wouldn't be in worse trouble.

After all, I told myself, we must wait for the results of tomorrow's catheterization to really know the whole truth.

First, we could safely assume because of the results of the PETscan that my coronary artery disease had progressed in some fashion. Secondly, we could not dismiss the heredity factor. Experts were agreed that heredity represented fifty percent of the cause of coronary disease, and it was the fifty percent you could do precious little about.

Another big cause of coronary disease was *hostility,* and in my case, it was one of the factors I had had little success in controlling.

I walked at a brisker pace and reminded myself that scientists were also busy adding another piece to the heart disease puzzle—cellular receptors that promote atherosclerosis (lesions in the arteries).

Investigators at the Massachusetts Institute of Technology had pinpointed cellular "receptors," modules that jut through a cell's surface and snag external chemicals and bring them into the cell.

The MIT scientists isolated two closely related scavenger receptors and the genes responsible for their formation.

Their work involved a lengthy purification of scavenger receptor molecules, enabling them to pinpoint the gene.

Soon, they should be able to control the growth of atherosclerotic lesions growing on my coronary arteries, I thought. After all, the pinpointing of the gene went right to the heart of the heredity problem, and it was, in all probability, the greatest advancement in treating atherosclerosis in the past decade.

I took a deep breath of sea air and quickened my pace. I was reminded that when my father died in the early 1940s, there was little treatment available for heart disease. Today, I was fortunate to have the advantages of angioplasty and the bypass operation as well as the benefits of modern drugs.

As I continued my fast-paced walk, it was clear to me how important understanding heredity's and hostility's contributions to heart disease were. Here I was feeling absolutely superb, walking as fast as my legs could carry me without the slightest fatigue. I had obviously conditioned my body to handle this physical exertion and my heart was so strong, it would not make the slightest complaint unless it was suddenly unable to receive even a portion of the blood it needed to operate.

This is why my treadmill and nuclear stress tests had been so successful. This is why they reported I was free of heart disease. I did not have the physical ability to tire my well-conditioned body to the point of exhaustion that would reveal the advancement of the atherosclerotic lesions on my coronaries. This was, obviously, why active people, convinced they were at the peak of good health, suddenly dropped dead without warning from a heart attack.

As I continued digging my feet into the sand, pushing myself with vigor toward the end of my walk, it became crystal clear to me that my program to keep my coronary artery disease under control had not been a failure. In fact, it had been a success—just not a perfect success.

If I had not committed the time and energy to the research I had done over the past two and a half years, I would not have known about the importance of a diagnostic tool such as the PETscan, and I would not have been motivated to

the point necessary to stay on top of my disease and anticipate its advancement.

My God, I thought, what the hell was I grumbling
about? My heart was still in perfect shape. It had not been
damaged or destroyed by a heart attack, and here I was
walking this earth with sufficient warning that there was a
high probability I would die from a massive heart attack
within weeks, certainly within months, if something wasn't
done about it.

In that thought lay the key. Something could be done
about it, and my self-education on heart disease permitted
me to make an informed choice of what could and must be
done.

I stopped. Looked heavenward, and thanked God for
the knowledge to anticipate the threat to my life and the
know-how to do something about it.

I *had* fallen into the one-third category. I wasn't one of
the two out of three whose coronary disease was stopped in
its tracks by the program I was on. But, because of the program, I had my life-saving warning, and now the thing to do
was not to, as Mom use to say, drench myself in a big dose of
PLOM (poor little ol' me). The thing to do was return to
Jacksonville that afternoon and undergo the catheterization
the following morning to reevaluate the growth of my coronary lesions, and use the talents of Drs. Onkar Narula and
David Hess to lay out a plan of action to deal with the problem.

Suddenly, I felt grateful to have learned of the advancement of my coronary disease in time to do something about
it. Anger, and self-pity really had no place in my thoughts.

My walking pace quickened even more as I headed
home, home to Jo to tell her what I was feeling, how I now
realized how fortunate I was to know, to be in position to do
something to save my life.

By late afternoon the next day, Dr. David Hess had performed the catheterization. It confirmed the PETscan's find-
ings, and, following six hours of bed rest, the punctures in

my groin where the catheters had been inserted were healed
sufficiently for me to get up.

Dr. Hess entered the room. "Let's go look at some pictures, Jay," he said.

I got out of bed, put my street clothes on, and Jo and I
followed him out of the room and down the hall. I was surprised that I had no feeling whatsoever from the catheterization. It was as if my body had not been touched. I felt as well
as I had the day before.

We followed Dr. Hess into a small room where my catheterization films were threaded in a projector and we spent
the next few minutes studying the lesions on my coronary
arteries.

We were joined by Dr. Donald Gordon, and both physicians told me the time had come to deal with my coronary
artery disease.

It was obvious that the situation was serious. It was obvious that I was running a risk that at any minute those
upper lesions could close and I would face a massive heart
attack with little hope of surviving.

Both physicians suggested I see Dr. Spencer King III at
Emory University's famed angioplasty department.

"Dr. Spencer King did my father's angioplasty, Jay. He
is among the best, if not *the* best angioplasty technician in
the country," Dr. Hess told me. "My father's disease was
about as advanced as yours and he's fine."

"I'm all for it," I said. "Something's gotta' be done."

"I'll set up the appointment," Dr. Hess smiled. "You go
up to Emory, they're super," he assured me. "They'll take
care of you."

I turned to Jo. She nodded affirmatively.

TWENTY-ONE

"The Decision"

Emory University Hospital sits in the rolling Druid Hills east of Atlanta, a typical university setting, but that's where typicality ends.

Inside the 604-bed medical complex Emory ranks as one of the busiest and most successful cardiac centers in the country, with extensive experience in evaluating the role of revascularization—the art of restoring blood flow to the heart.

More than 15,000 patients have received coronary artery bypass surgery in its cardiac care units, and the Health Care Financing Administration, the federal agency which operates the Medicare program, reports Emory hospitals have one of the nation's lowest mortality figures. But most importantly to me, the center is a leader in the treatment of all heart disease, especially angioplasty.

The technique of opening the coronary arteries with a balloon was developed at Emory by Dr. Andreas Gruentzig, who was unfortunately killed in a plane crash in 1985.

Today, Emory's Gruentzig Cardiovascular Center is in the capable hands of Dr. Spencer B. King III, professor of medicine (cardiology) and radiology.

As soon as Jo and I arrived, I clearly knew Emory was where I should be. Minutes after passing through the admitting office gates, we were met by a pleasant staff in the

Gruentzig Center, and then Dr. Nicholas J. Lembo invited Jo and me into his office for a background briefing.

Dr. Lembo told us a team of Emory physicians had been selected by the National Institute of Health to receive an $8 million grant to determine if angioplasty is as effective and safe a therapy for patients with multivessel coronary artery disease as coronary bypass surgery.

"It sounds like I'm a prime candidate for the study," I told him.

"That's what I wanted to talk to you about," he said. "I'll give you the facts about both treatments and we'll take it from there."

"What you are saying is I have a choice between angioplasty and bypass surgery?"

"Not exactly," he smiled.

"Whatta' you mean?"

"If you decide to enter the study, the computer will select your treatment," he said.

Like hell it will, I thought. I'll select my own treatment. I was suddenly somewhat aghast. I had been sent to Emory to undergo angioplasty, and now I was being told I could have either bypass surgery or the balloon dilation.

"I thought Drs. Hess and King agreed I should have the angioplasty?" I questioned.

"Not necessarily," Dr. Lembo explained. "For the past twenty-five years, bypass surgery has been the standard treatment for your disease." He went on to explain that in my case, after he and Dr. King had studied my catheterization films, they'd decided that I had a choice between bypass surgery and angioplasty.

Dr. Lembo also explained that even though I was a good candidate for the National Institute of Health study, the number of lesions on my left anterior descending coronary artery did not make me a good patient for either bypass or angioplasty.

What I had going for me was Emory itself. I was in *the* medical center where some of the country's top cardiac experts practiced, and I felt the best that could be done for me would be done in these facilities.

This was a comforting thought in spite of my predicament, and Jo and I sat there listening intently to Dr. Lembo tell us that the coronary artery bypass graft surgery would involve use of the internal mammary artery to my left anterior descending coronary and possibly a saphenous vein graft.

Dr. Lembo said the bypass operation usually involves being in the hospital for six or seven days and then four to six week recovery period. He added that the major risks of bypass surgery include myocardial infarction (heart attack), stroke, infection, and death.

"We think that the chance for any one of these events occuring would probably be less than two percent in your case, Mr. Barbree."

"Is that average?" I asked.

"Yes," he answered.

"What is the risk for angioplasty?"

"About the same," he smiled. "As I said, you should benefit from either."

Dr. Lembo added, the negative aspects of surgery are that it involves a major operation with all the risks associated with that, and if reoperation is needed in the future, the risk is some four- to five-fold higher for a second operation.

"But in spite of the risks, hasn't bypass surgery for my condition been a standard procedure?" I asked.

"That's correct," he said, adding, "and we have very skilled surgeons here.

"So I understand," I nodded. "Tell me about angioplasty."

"Well," he took a breath before beginning. "Angioplasty involves placing a small balloon in the area of the blockage through a catheter placed in the leg." He went on to explain that the balloon is then advanced to the site of the blockage and then inflated. This is successful in approximately ninety-five percent of patients, but, he cautioned, there are two major drawbacks with angioplasty. There is approximately a three to four percent chance that while doing the angioplasty, the artery does not stay open and in fact becomes occluded and emergency bypass surgery is needed. Emergency bypass surgery is probably needed in approximately two to three percent of patients who have single vessel coronary disease.

"The likelihood of emergency bypass surgery for me because of my multivessel disease would be much higher, wouldn't it?"

"Yes," he nodded, "much higher."

I glanced at Jo. Her eyes met mine. Sometimes words are not necessary.

Dr. Lembo continued, telling us that emergency bypass surgery brought on by a collapsing artery caused by angioplasty is usually more risky that elective bypass surgery because the patient is going to the operating room in the presence of limitation of blood flow to the heart—in some cases during a heart attack itself.

Dr. Lembo explained that during an emergency bypass the surgeon generally is unable to use the mammary artery —today's preferred artery for a bypass—because it takes some forty-five minutes to an hour to prepare the mammary for use.

What makes the mammary artery bypass so effective is that the arteries, which supply the breasts with blood, are located just above the heart. Because of this, the internal mammary, usually the left one, is not cut away from the position it was placed in by nature. It is simply rerouted to bypass the blockage and sewn to the coronary artery farther downstream.

Twelve to fifteen years after a mammary bypass (the total history of the mammary operation), ninety-five percent of the mammary arteries are still open. Because the mammary is very much like a coronary artery, it is the best bypass operation available today.

A major drawback with angioplasty is restenosis. Restenosis, Dr. Lembo told us, is when the blockage which was dilated by the balloon reoccurs. This happens in about thirty percent of the patients who have one vessel blocked. This event normally takes place in the first six months after angioplasty, and the patient needs to come back again for a repeat angioplasty.

"Again," I interrupted, "the likelihood I would need to repeat the angioplasty is much higher for me, correct?"

"Correct," he answered. "Because you have several blockages."

"So, the question is," I asked, "are the lesions on my left anterior descending artery suitable for angioplasty?"

"Correct," he nodded. "We have done over ten thousand angioplasty procedures here at Emory." He added confidently, "We're prepared to do yours."

"If the computer selects angioplasty for me," I grinned.

"That's correct."

"And if I join your study."

"Again, correct," he smiled.

"Tell me more."

"Well, what the study is trying to learn," he began, "is whether patients with multivessel disease, such as yourself, should undergo angioplasty or should continue to undergo coronary artery bypass grafting.

"So far, we have enrolled close to four hundred patients in the study," he smiled. "Half went to surgery, the other half went to angioplasty."

"But they didn't have a choice," I stated.

"No," he shook his head. "It's important for the computer to select each patient's treatment. That way," he explained, "we should have an equal and fair result from the study."

"Anything else?"

"Yes," he said. "All patients enrolled in the study are asked to return here at one and three year intervals from their procedure and undergo a cardiac catheterization and a thallium stress test."

"The catheterization adds an additional risk, doesn't it?"

He smiled. "Not with Drs. King and Douglas doing them."

I nodded. "They're that good, huh?"

"That good," he nodded in agreement.

"Well, this one I've gotta' think about," I told him. "When do you need an answer?"

"First," he said, "let me introduce you to Dr. King, and later today, when he is through with his scheduled surgery, I would like you to meet and talk with one of our best surgeons, Dr. Joe Craver.

"Then, I can give you my answer?"

"Sure," he smiled, "but Dr. Craver is going to recommend surgery."

"What do you recommend?"

"Well," he said, "your multi-lesion disease in one vessel makes you a candidate for our government study. I think you would benefit from either procedure."

"Aw, come on, Dr. Lembo," I smiled. "Think of me as your favorite uncle. Which one would you recommend for him?"

He grinned. "My answer would have to be the same."

"Okay," I laughed, moving toward the door.

We went into the hallway where we could see three men talking in a room across the hall.

"There's Dr. King," Dr. Lembo said, leading us into the room, and Jo and I were introduced to the professor.

We exchanged pleasantries and, I must admit, I stood before the slim, somewhat shy man in awe.

Not only did Dr. Spencer B. King III project quiet confidence, the professor looked like a taller, younger Jimmy Carter and commanded from those in the room the same respect as the former president.

"Has Dr. Lembo explained our government study?" Dr. King asked.

"Yes, quite well," I answered.

"We've studied your catheterization, Jay," he said, reaching for a roll of 35mm film on a shelf above his head, "and your case presents us with somewhat of a problem."

"I didn't plan it that way," I smiled.

"I understand," he said, placing the film in a nearby projector. "You see," he continued as the film rolled and we could see the dye rushing through my left anterior descending artery, "you have these sequential lesions beginning at the top of the vessel."

"Yes, sir," I acknowledged.

"These lesions seem to run together," he explained. "They take up pretty much the top half of the artery."

I stared at the film. God, I thought. That's a sickly looking vessel. Its eaten alive with lesions, and the real question was, was it worth repairing? But, I knew, there was only one answer. If I were to live, blood flow had to be restored.

Dr. King invited Jo and me into his office where we continued the conversation.

"What are the facts, Dr. King?" I asked. "What are my real odds?

"Jay," he began. "I think I can help you," he said without solid confidence, "but there's a seven to eight percent chance you'll have to have emergency bypass surgery."

"And?"

"And, if we are successful with angioplasty," he answered, "there's a forty-five percent chance you'll have to come back and have us do it again."

"Fifty-fifty," I said quietly.

"Fifty-fifty," he repeated.

I settled back in my chair. My condition was now most clear to me, and it was also most clear that I had a tough decision to make. I knew it was time for me to do some serious evaluating, to do some serious praying, to ask God to help me make the right decision.

I spent the afternoon with a legal-size yellow pad in my hands, jotting down the pros and cons of angioplasty versus surgery. I summoned every fact I had learned about the subject as if my life depended on it. The sad truth was it did, and I began by first running the facts about bypass surgery through my mind.

The procedure had been performed hundreds of thousands of times during the past quarter of a century, and some critics were saying surgeons were performing a large number of the operations when they were not needed.

But I also knew that, unlike bypass surgery, there are no rigid training requirements for performing coronary angioplasty. Any cardiologist trained in heart catheterization can go through a two-week angioplasty training course, buy the equipment and set up shop, unsupervised, in a hospital. And unlike surgery, there are no watchdogs. A single cardiologist often evaluates, tests and performs angioplasty on a patient.

Anyone who is considering the procedure at a hospital other than the major centers like Emory should ask their doctor a few key questions.

The first, of course, should be, "How many angioplasties have you done?"

The Society for Cardiac Angiography and Interventions (SCA) recommends a minimum of one hundred twenty-five procedures during training and at least fifty a year thereafter. But many experts believe a practitioner should do at least two a week to keep skills well honed.

The second question would be, "What percentage of your patients have a heart attack, die or suffer a complication during the procedure requiring surgery?"

In centers such as Emory one to two percent of angioplasty patients die, 4.3 percent suffer a heart attack and 3.4 percent require emergency bypass surgery. If the numbers are higher where you are, have the procedure done elsewhere.

The third question should be, "Will there by a surgery team standing by in case of an emergency?"

It's mandatory, in case a vessel is punctured or a heart attack occurs during angioplasty; and, if the doctor doing the diagnosis is going to perform the angioplasty, get a second opinion.

I was also reminding myself that in a bypass operation, the results are more final. You don't have to go back for a redo. But, I was also reminding myself, neither angioplasty nor bypass surgery cures heart disease. Only a regimen that incorporates diet, exercise, low cholesterol, and a hostility-free attitude can reduce risk.

The biggest argument in favor of angioplasty was that if the procedure was successful, you would be over it in a couple of days. The biggest argument against bypass was that if it was successful, you would need two to six months to really get over the cutting through of your breastbone and muscles and tendons and flesh.

"Yuuuuukkkkkkkkk," I let out a Bronx cheer. Neither alternative was all that appealing, but the real challenge for me was to come to a decision that would offer the most permanent solution.

The afternoon passed and the darkness of evening had arrived and I was back in Dr. Kings office when a tall, strong man dressed in surgical greens came through the door. Before Dr. Lembo could speak, I felt the need to rise to my feet, not to waste this man's time.

"Jay, this is Dr. Joe Craver."

I lifted my right hand, grasping his, feeling a firm grip.

"I'm sorry to be late," he said, "but I've just finished my fifth operation today."

"No problem, no reason to apologize," I sputtered. "What you were doing was far more important than this."

He nodded and turned to face Jo as Dr. Lembo introduced my wife and, with the social formalities out of the way, we went into the room where my catheterization films were loaded in the projector.

The physicians studied my diseased coronaries and when they were through we settled in Dr. Lembo's office.

"Son," Dr. Craver began in his soft, comfortable North Carolina accent, "I understand Dr. Lembo has told you about his government program?"

"Yes, sir, he has."

"Well," he said flatly. "You gotta' get something done. That left anterior artery of yours is in pretty bad shape."

"Yes sir."

"The plaque starts up at the top and seems to continue almost in one unbroken lesion, instead of the three that are there."

I nodded, acknowledging I understood.

"So, whatta' you gonna' do?" he asked bluntly.

"Well, I can tell you what I'm not gonna' do," I smiled. "I'm not gonna' let a computer select my treatment."

Dr. Craver grinned.

"I've been trying to get Dr. Lembo to give me his opinion, but he won't tell me," I laughed. "Not even if I was his favorite uncle."

"You didn't asked me my opinion," Dr. Craver said bluntly, surprising me and startling Dr. Lembo.

"Good, Lord," I sputtered again, "of course I want your opinion Dr. Craver. I just thought you wouldn't . . ."

"Surgery," he interrupted.

"Surgery?"

"Surgery, son," he said clearly. "You're not a good candidate for angioplasty."

"I'm not?"

"No, sir," he answered with full confidence. "That plaque has probably calcified in your artery and angioplasty just won't get the job done, son."

"What about the problem of sewing a graft to my artery between the lesions?"

"Hell, son," he said with his can-do attitude, "if I just drop your left internal mammary artery down past those upper lesions I've done you a whole lotta' good."

"Dr. King says there's a forty-five percent chance I'll have to come back if his angioplasty is successful."

"Oh, you'll have to come back," Dr. Craver said.

I nodded I understood and added, "And there's almost a one in ten chance you'll have to perform bypass surgery on me anyway."

"Right."

I stood up. "When can you do it?"

"Not tomorrow, son," he said. "I'm going hunting tomorrow. I'll do you the first thing Thursday morning. You'll be the first in. You won't have to wait."

I felt energized, "That's great. Let's do it!."

Jo looked a little startled, but she knew I had made my decision. And as always was ready to support me even though earlier, she had been leaning toward the angioplasty with the thought we would be out of there in a couple of days.

"You'd better ask him what he's going to charge you," Dr. Lembo spoke up, "before you make a final decision."

I waved a hand. "I don't care about that," I said. "My union, AFTRA (American Federation of Television and Radio Artists), has its members covered up to a million dollars."

"Half of that will do me," Dr. Craver laughed.

"You can have it," I returned the laughter, "if you take care of my problem."

I suddenly felt sorry for Dr. Lembo. He had been so nice to us, had taken a lot of time with us to explain his program and the benefits of both treatments, and I had quickly and absolutely made my decision to go with surgery.

I turned to him. "I really appreciate all the time you've taken with us, Dr. Lembo, but I'd like to get this problem behind me," I explained. "Surgery offers that. Angioplasty could be a never-ending treatment."

He nodded. "I understand. You had a tough decision to make."

"Thank you," I said, turning to walk with Dr. Craver to the door and into the hallway where I suddenly had him alone.

"I appreciate you taking me as patient, Dr. Craver," I told the surgeon. "I certainly hope you can do me some good."

He stopped, faced me. "Son," he began in a Burt Reynolds sort of manner, "you are not a good candidate for angioplasty. You made your only decision."

"I feel I have."

"Dr. Spencer King is the best there is at it," he explained, "but there's not much of a chance they can reopen those calcified lesions of yours, not all of 'em."

I nodded agreement.

"Now, I'll get with Dr. King, and we'll study your films again," he continued. "We'll look for a clean spot in your artery where I can sew your internal mammary artery between the lesions, do what we call a sequential bypass."

"I hope my mammary artery will be long enough to do the job," I smiled. "I hope you don't have to use a vein."

He put his hand on my shoulder. "Heck, son," he said, "as tall as you are your mammary should be plenty long. We shouldn't have a problem."

"That'll be just great," I smiled.

"Don't worry, son," he said, walking away. "We'll take care of you."

I watched the tall surgeon stride confidently down the hallway. I was instantly aware that I had just put my fate in his hands. And the best part of it was that I felt good about it, felt confident myself. I sensed in Dr. Joe Craver that can-do attitude I had long associated with the astronauts. There was in the man a confidence that there wasn't a mountain too high for him to climb, a sea too broad for him to cross. Dr. Joe Craver was my kind of man. When there was a difficult job to be done, he simply went out and did it.

I couldn't help but think about the lives he had saved, sense his efforts to be the best at what he did, and I stood there thankful he had agreed to put those talents to work in my behalf.

TWENTY-TWO

"The Day Before"

That Wednesday, the day before my operation, was, for the first time since my PETscan exam two weeks before, worry-free. It was a day spent getting ready. A day being visited by Dr. Craver's assistants who asked pages after pages of questions while technicians worked over my body drawing blood, taking X-rays, taking my temperature and searching for any evidence of the presence of an illness.

I was fascinated by the medical tests as well as the questions, and I spent the day confident I was ready to put my body in the shop for repairs.

Charlotte, Dr. King's secretary, called and Jo and I went up to his office where we found him studying my catheterization films, getting ready to make his recommendations to Dr. Craver. He was looking for a clean spot in my diseased anterior descending coronary where Dr. Craver could splice in the mammary artery to bypass the upper lesions. If this could be done, then Dr. Craver could loop the mammary around a seventy percent blockage downstream and terminate the mammary artery beyond the disease.

Dr. King explained this would give the lower half of my heart a good blood supply and should take care of the problem Dr. Donald Gordon had found in my PETscan.

It was not enough just to see and guess at the amount of blockage revealed by the cardiac catheterization, it was im-

259

portant to know the amount of blood flow reaching every cell of the heart muscle. PETscan told you that.

What I found fascinating was the advancement, or lack of advancement of the coronary artery disease itself. "Dr. King, that seventy percent lesion you are concerned about getting that sequential bypass around," I said, pointing, "has been seventy percent ever since I had my first catheterization in 1977."

"Your dieting, exercise, and other efforts," he answered, "have stabilized that one."

"And the one on my circumflex artery hasn't progressed since my catheterization in Miami two and a half years ago," I continued, "and some of this plaque along my anterior descending appears to have reversed itself."

"It could have," he smiled. "Though these upper lesions have advanced, your new lifestyle has had an effect on the rest of your coronary disease."

That statement by the professor made me feel better. It was additional evidence that the job of fighting coronary artery disease is a complicated one, and that it was a job of not only lowering your cholesterol, it was a job of using all the other elements possible such as exercise and, most importantly, an anger-free attitude.

I was very grateful for the effort Dr. King was making on my behalf. After all I had chosen the bypass operation instead of his angioplasty, but, regardless of my decision, here was this outstanding authority on heart disease giving his time to help make sure the operation was a success.

That evening, I found many more people in my corner. Minister Ray Goolsby and his father Henry (our builder), called my room and prayed for me over the phone.

And at the same time, in south Georgia, my sisters Billie, Jean, and Lois were praying while touching a picture of me holding my grandson, Bryce.

Son Steve in Illinois included me in his prayers as did daughters Alicia and Karla in Florida.

I didn't feel the least bit alone, and I wasn't. About eight o'clock I got shaved all over (this time by a man), and I showered twice with a special soap to cleanse my body of germs.

Jo decided to spend the evening in my room by sleeping in a fold-down chair, and I never felt more at ease, more ready.

Years before I had learned a very important lesson in a very graphic way during an aircraft descent into San Diego's Lindbergh Field.

A group of us reporters from the Cape were on an Air Force tour of facilities on the West Coast, and while flying from one space facility to another, we spent the time playing penny-ante poker.

I was seated by the window, flying backwards, and it was my turn to deal. We were on our final approach into Lindbergh, with all the losers crying.

I glanced out the window and was surprised to see how low we were flying over the tops of TV antenna-laden roofs. "Hey, look at this," I said excitedly, pointing. "We're getting real close to those houses."

Colonel Ken Grine, our escort and a no nonsense kind of guy, stared at me impatiently. "Can you do anything about it?"

"Nope," I said.

"Well, deal," he cried. "I'm down nearly two dollars."

Oh, another thing about my friend Ken Grine, he's not only impatient, he's cheap, but, more importantly, he was right; his point made a lasting impression on me.

The aircraft was in the hands of the crew.

Now I felt the same emotions I felt then. My future was in the hands of Emory's professionals and the Man upstairs. There was no reason for worry.

I never felt more at ease, more ready.

Relax, Jay, I told myself. You're just along for the ride.

TWENTY-THREE

"The Operation"

For a long time I lay between sleep and coming awake, hesitant to leave that in-between mood of looseness. Jo had slept with her body stretched uncomfortably across the fold-down chair, not with her body snuggling close to mine as it had for so many years. But even without our familiar and comfortable togetherness, I drifted off again, coming awake a second time to the sound of voices. The nurses, I thought, and then I heard the laughter of happy people going about their work. The sound was drifting in soft echoes through the hospital room door and I thought of it as a nice sound. Once, long ago, I used to keep a collection of special, pleasant sounds in my mind. Remembering it now, I added this one.

I stirred under the blanket and turned to look at Jo, drawing comfort from the fact she was there, but realizing what an uncomfortable night it had to have been for her. Again, I simply did not expect her to be anywhere else. We were partners, we were bunkies, and I knew she would be there every moment that day, ready to help in any way to make sure my mammary artery bypass operation went well as planned.

I clasped my hands together and looked up, thanking God for another day, and as my mind cleared, it cleared with the realization that I was lying in the hospital bed, ready to have the blood flow to my heart restored because of my self-management health program.

The evidence from the University of Southern California study and others suggested the program was successful in two out of three cases, and the addition of surgery, or balloon angioplasty, or a number of other corrective techniques, offered success for the third case.

As part of the program, the PETscan exam caught the life-threatening blockage even though my efforts at controlling my cholesterol, staying on a proper diet, and exercising correctly, stabilized the remainder of my coronary artery disease, and even reversed some lesions.

The clarity of morning also brought with it the understanding that possibly the reason that God had permitted my life to be restored on the beach May 27th, 1987 was for me, as a communicator, to communicate the success of such a self-management health program.

The fact that I had drawn the more ominous third straw, the one person in three for whom the program did not completely arrest all of the growth of coronary artery disease, simply meant that the program had done its job by bringing me to Emory for corrective action.

The results of the program that had brought me to the operating table reminded me of the story of John, the Christian whose home was caught in a major flood.

John sat on his front porch watching the water rise, and when a boat came to pick him up, he refused to leave, saying "The Lord will provide."

He even refused the help of a second boat when the rising water forced him onto the roof, and when he was standing on the last dry part of the top of the house, a helicopter came and he gave the same reply: "The Lord will provide."

The helicopter flew away and a few minutes later John was washed away. As he drowned, he asked, "Why have you forsaken me, Lord?"

A silent answer swept loudly through his mind. I sent you two boats and a helicopter, John, what more would you have me do?

Of course, the point of the story is too many people

depend too much on God and on others to provide supernatural aid for them when, if they simply looked around them, there are God given natural opportunities for the taking.

The sounds of groans came from Jo's direction and my early morning thoughts were interrupted by watching her stretch her arms above her head, trying to free her body of the cramps and aches brought on by sleeping on that fold-down chair.

"Morning," she said.

"Comfortable?" I replied.

She frowned and sat up, yawning and stretching her body more before managing to move into the bathroom where she brushed her teeth and washed her face.

"How do you feel?" she asked, standing in the door.

"Wonderful," I smiled. "It's a good morning for it."

"Nervous?"

"Not a bit," I answered. "I couldn't be more ready."

"You'd better be," a grinning nurse said as she entered the room. "You're the first up."

"I'm number one on the runway, huh?"

"Yep," she said. "I've got something for you."

The nurse handed me a small tablet and a cup with water. "Take only a small sip," she instructed, "just enough to get it down. Don't want anything coming up during surgery."

"What is it?"

"Valium."

"Uh huh."

"I've got something else," she smiled, lifting a fully loaded hyperdermic needle.

"Is that my 'I don't care' shot?"

"Something like that," she grinned.

"Let me brush my teeth first," I pleaded.

"That's not necessary."

"Please," I said, I renewed my plea. "I don't want to blast the operating team with bad breath."

She and Jo laughed out loud.

"Go ahead," the nurse chuckled, "But you'll have so much stuff in your throat they'll never smell it."

I didn't answer. I litterly leaped from the bed and grabbed my tooth brush. "Joooooo," I mumbled through the pasty foam and brush strokes, "makeeee sureee youuuu packkkk allllll myyyyy stufffff."

"I'll take care of everything, Jay," she said. "You get back in bed," she laughed again. "I wanna' see you take your shot."

"Meany," I grumbled, sipping water to wash the tooth paste from my mouth.

"Don't swallow any of that," the nurse instructed.

"I didn't," I assured her, returning to bed and to the needle.

I rolled over on my side and felt the needle penetrate the flesh of my upper buttocks. Morphine to reduce the discomfort of the necessary needle sticks, mixed with scopolamine, an added sedative which would give me a dry mouth, flowed into my flesh and blood and, with the aid of the valium, I began to feel drowsy within minutes.

Jo sat quietly and I let the medications work. There was no reason to talk. Everything that could be said had been said, and my wife knew I was ready for the surgery. That, was really, the only surprise of the morning. I had thought if the day ever came that I would need major surgery, I would be more anxious, more up tight about the fact people were about to cut open my body, to literally reach inside and hold my heart in their hands. Well, I wasn't, and I attributed that to the fact I understood what had to be done, and I was most grateful it would be done by some of the best in the country. I laughed. Remember the landing at Lindbergh Field in San Diego. There's not a thing you can do about it. Relax.

I did, and they came for me with a rolling bed, and Jo ran around, nervous, making sure she had gathered all our belongings because we would not be returning to the same room.

I said a sleepy goodbye to her and the nurse and we were on our way down what seemed like many hallways and a couple of elevators until we reached what they called the holding area outside of the operating room.

I began to drift in and out of sleep, occasionally aware that needles were being stuck in my arms and I was being moved about, being positioned for the operation. It was an atmosphere of trust, a sleepy scene of being with and in the hands of very nice, competent people.

Emory University Hospital's operating room #4 is engineering and life sciences frontis piece wrapped up in a gleaming high-tech package. It has the latest in equipment, the latest in human knowhow, and is one of the places where lives are literally saved, where years in a single life are added—years that are only a blink of a universal instant, but another lifetime to a Jay Barbree and to all the others who are seeking to continue their lives, to spend a few more years with family and with friends and with jobs and with community needs.

There were men and women there for the reporter's operation who were at the forefront of late twentieth century medicine. Men and women who knew as much about flesh and blood and sinew and tendon and muscle and bones and marrow and veins and arteries and nerves and pulsing liquid flow and of trillions of cells as could be known on November 30th, 1989.

One among them, Dr. John Waller, professor and chairman of Emory's anesthesiology department, stared at the patient.

"This guy's LTBA (lucky to be alive)," he said to the others. "He had cardiac arrest while jogging," he added. "Anyone who can survive that should have no trouble getting through a little heart surgery."

Barbree opened sleepy eyes. "A piece of cake," he managed to smile.

Dr. Waller and the others laughed and the professor began readying the patient for the operation.

Anesthesiology resident Dr. David Wimberly had already positioned Jay on the operating table and had placed two large-bore IV's into his arm veins. Dr. Waller scrubbed the right side of his neck, placed a sterile drape over the area, and through a "numb spot" made by injecting a local anesthetic, he inserted a pulmonary artery catheter into Jay's internal jugular vein. This long, yellow plastic catheter containing multiple channels passes through the right side of the heart

*and into position in the pulmonary artery, the main blood
vessel from the heart to the lungs. When connected to the
computer and electronic pressure measuring devices, it provides important information on a continuous basis about the
performance of the cardiovascular system.*

*With this procedure complete and all monitors and ma-
chines checked and calibrated, Dr. Waller was ready to administer the anesthetic drugs to put Barbree to sleep.*

*"Jay, we're ready to begin," he told the patient. "Are you
comfortable?"*

*"Tell you what," a sleepy Barbree replied, "why don't I
just sit up and watch the whole thing?"*

"I'm afraid that won't work," Dr. Waller laughed.

"You've been wonderful," Barbree said. "I love you all."

*The surgical team looked at each other, smiling, and Dr.
Waller administered the drug Midazolam through the IV tub-
ing, and the reporter drifted off to sleep breathing pure oxygen
through a mask.*

*A few minutes later the anesthetic vapor Enflurane was
added to the oxygen Barbree breathed to help maintain his
anesthetized state. Dr. Waller adjusted the breathing mixture
moment to moment to balance the physiologic demands of
surgery and the everchanging status of the reporter's cardiovascular system. Another drug, Vecuronium, was administered to cause temporary muscle paralysis, necessary to permit opening the chest and exposing the heart to the surgeon.
Dr. Waller knew use of this drug literally placed Barbree's life
in his and the surgical team's hands because he would be
unable to breathe, totally depending on those in the operating
room to do so for him. Fentanyl, a synthetic narcotic drug one
hundred times more potent than morphine, was given at intervals to complete the anesthetic. This drug blocked normal
but potentially harmful responses to the pain of surgery,
which could occur even when the patient was unconscious.
An endotracheal (breathing) tube was placed into Barbree's
trachea, and was connected to a mechanical ventilator. This
machine provided the reporter's every breath for many hours
thereafter, except for the interval when the heart-lung machine did the work.*

Meanwhile an electrosurgical grounding pad was placed under Barbree's buttocks and the surgical team scrubbed his body with skin cleanser before painting him with a betadine solution from his neck to his ankles. His red body was then covered with sterile drapes, and a large table holding the instruments and supplies was placed over the patient's feet.

The team was good, the surgeons incredible. One doctor, Joseph Craver, had long ago moved through most coronary bypass surgery and beyond, and once again he was ready to attempt to repair a body.

Dr. Craver and his team's creed was simple. It was the work itself, and they began by cutting through the skin of the chest from two inches below the neck to four inches above the navel. An air-driven saw was then used to cut through the tough bone and cartilage and gristle that is the sternum, and a large retractor was placed in the chest. The instrument was cranked open to expose the pericardium (the lining that protects the heart).

The heart's lining was opened with an electrosurgical knife, and sutures were placed in the pericardium to spread it open, exposing the heart muscle itself.

With the heart exposed, Heparin (to prevent temporarily the normal process of blood clotting) was given and the surgeons placed large tubes for the heart-lung (cardiopulmonary bypass) machine into his heart and aorta.

The heart-lung machine was turned on and Dr. Waller turned off the ventilator so that Barbree's lungs stopped moving. His blood now circulated through the heart-lung machine, named because it served both as his lungs (removing carbon dioxide and adding oxygen) and as his heart (mechanically providing blood pressure). This permitted the reporter's own heart to be stopped with a potassium-rich solution to immobilize it for the operation.

Opening the chest and placing him on the heart-lung bypass machine proceeded rapidly, and then the surgical team harvested Jay Barbree's left internal mammary artery.

The internal mammary arteries supply blood to the breasts and, because of their location near the heart, they are very much akin to the coronary arteries themselves. This makes the mammary the most desired artery to be used as a graft around a coronary artery blockage, plus they do not have to be cut away from where they naturally branch off from a larger artery just inches above the heart itself. The mammary is simply rerouted from the breast to form a anastomosis (two ends going together) with the coronary to bypass the blockage.

To protect his heart and other vital organs during the operation, his body temperature was lowered to 28 degrees C., and a cross-clamp was used to clamp the aorta shut to isolate the heart from any blood flow.

Next a 14 gauge angiocatheter was placed in the aorta below the cross-clamp to perfuse the heart and the coronary arteries with cardioplegia (called "magic"). Cardioplegia is used to preserve the myocardium (the muscular substance of the heart) while the cross-clamp is on.

Dr. Joe Craver now literally held Jay Barbree's heart in his hands and he studied the left anterior descending artery, the diseased vessel. He could see and feel it was made rigid by atherosclerotic lesions and calcified in its proximal half.

"Someone is watching over this guy," he said quietly. "He made the right decision. Angioplasty would've never worked."

The skilled surgeon searched for a soft spot in the diseased artery, finding it in the mid-portion of the vessel where he used very small, continuous running sutures to create a side-to-side mammary anastomosis with the left anterior descending artery.

Dr. Craver then took a 1.5 mm probe and pushed it through the anastomosis down to the junction of the mid and distal third of the vessel where it would go no farther. It was being blocked by the seventy percent lesion that had been discovered twelve years earlier, but had been stabilized by Barbree's diet and exercise program.

Dr. Craver decided to use the mammary artery to skip over the lesion and he created a second anastomosis end to side with the bypass artery.

When the cross-clamp was removed from the aorta, there was excellent flow in the mammary artery in both these areas and it promptly filled the diseased anterior descending coronary artery and all its branches with bright, red blood.

The surgeons smiled, and the patient was allowed to rest for a while before the blood flowing through the heart-lung machine was warmed to normal body temperature.

Barbree's heart began to beat spontaneously when the warmed blood reached the new coronary bypasses, a good sign at that point in the operation.

A patient with a badly damaged heart might require almost heroic treatment with powerful drugs and mechanical devices to make his heart strong enough to resume its lifelong function of pumping life-sustaining blood to the body. In the worst cases, the doctors can't make that happen.

But Jay Barbree was being brought off the heart-lung machine without the need for cardiovascular support drugs to stimulate his heart. He was in excellent condition and sinus rhythm. Everything looked good as the artificial circulation was discontinued, and normal blood flow through the reporter's own heart and lungs was restored without any problem.

Before surgery, Barbree's heart was strong and his operation had proceeded without incident. This demonstrated how important preventive medicine programs were, how important it was to anticipate trouble and take care of it before damage occurs.

Jay Barbree came to surgery with a strong, undamaged heart, and he was leaving it the same way.

*J*o Barbree sat out the operation in the Cardiac Intensive Care waiting room with others waiting to learn the fate of family members undergoing surgery. It was time spent in a sort of slow motion, an inner focus that left room for little of the outside world. It was time spent while the skills of others repaired the handiwork of God, extended life, or, if the skills failed, finished it.

She knew the outcome would mean a major change in her life. It would mean a renewal, another rebirth for her husband, a new lease that would mean more years together, or it would. . . .

She didn't want to think about that! Instead, she stood

up, moved about the room, and checked her watch—10:30. Too early to hear anything, she thought. They said the operation would take four to five hours and Jay had been in there only three.

She started out into the hall when she heard the phone ring on the volunteer hospital worker's desk. Something told her to wait. She turned to see the lady listening on the phone, and she decided to sit back down. She had a feeling.

The hospital volunteer looked directly at her and smiled. "Mrs. Barbree, your husband is off the bypass machine."

Sudden relief swept through her. "That's wonderful," she said.

"That's the biggy," the volunteer explained. "That means his heart is beating on its own. He's through the operation."

"When can I see him?"

"Oh, he'll be in post-op for more than an hour," the lady said, "but they'll bring him down this hall, by the door here." She smiled. "You'll get to see him then."

Jo returned to her feet and time seem to return to its normal pace. All seem back in order. She was now fully confident Jay would make it. The surgeons had done their job, and if she knew her husband, he would breeze through recovery. After all he was the guy who they told would never be six feet tall because his mother was only five foot two, and his father stood five ten. But Jay was determined, and he made it with two inches to spare.

She laughed. Her six foot two husband. She was barely five four. Mutt and Jeff. The short and the tall of it! But it was a match that had lasted, and, now, thanks to the good Lord and a skillful Emory medical team, it appeared it would be a match that would last even longer.

Jo took up a post at the door to the hallway and began waiting again. Waiting this time for a hospital bed to come rolling by. Within only a few minutes, one did. But it wasn't her husband, and neither was the next, or the one after that.

She knew it was too early, but it seemed the thing to do, so she just waited. Waited more than an hour until a herd of hospital workers came rushing down the hallway with a bed supporting bags and tubes and all sort of medical equipment

*and she tried to see who was on it, but there were so many
people.*

*The rolling bed passed as quickly as it came and before it
got too far down the hall, she spotted a familiar crop of
golden, brown hair. She smiled. Jay's once auburn hair, now
bleached golden by days after days of walking on the beach.*

*She turned back to the hospital volunteer. "It's him," she
said. "He's on his way to Intensive Care."*

*"You should go for a walk, get something to eat, or some-
thing," the volunteer told her. "You won't be able to go in until
visiting hours."*

*Jo smiled. "First, I think I'll find a rest-room," she said,
walking away.*

*When she returned, she spotted Dr. Joseph Craver com-
ing out of one of the waiting rooms. "Mrs. Barbree," he called.
"Your husband is a champ," he smiled broadly. "He went
through the operation without a hitch. In fact," the enthusias-
tic surgeon continued, "we got through the whole thing in
about three hours."*

"He's okay?"

*"Oh, just great," Dr. Craver said. "He's got a strong heart.
It restarted on its own after the surgery."*

"What did you do?" she asked.

*"Oh," he grinned. "Just the mammary artery bypass—
two bypasses," he explained. "It worked great. Restored the
blood flow. There shouldn't be a problem."*

"You didn't have to take a vein out of his leg?"

*"Oh, no," Dr. Craver answered, shaking his head. "He's
so tall his mammary artery was nice and long and wide
open," he said, pointing. "That's important."*

*"Thank you, Dr. Craver," she said, watching the surgeon
walk away.*

*He slowed his pace and looked back over his shoulder.
"Remember," he called, "I want an invitation to come down
and see one of those night shuttle launches."*

"You got it, Dr. Craver," she waved. "Jay'll set it up."

*He returned the wave and vanished from her view. It
was great news, but it all seemed too quick. There was so
much more she had wanted to ask, but she knew how busy
Dr. Craver was. How much he was needed. And she also knew*

there was another friend her husband needed just as much. Time—time for the shock of the operation to dissipate from Jay's system, time for trillions of cells to re-form and to adjust to whatever additional years he had just been given.

TWENTY-FOUR

"The Recovery"

*B*RRRRRRRRRRRRRRRT!

I froze, startled by a sound I'd heard too many times in my life. An unmistakable sound. The machine-gun screech of the reptile world.

Heat and chills moved in waves up my back and sprouted with dampness on my face. I moved cautiously backward, every so slowly, and—

BRRRRRRRRRRRRRRRT!

There it was again! The sound of warning and fury coiled at the end of a giant mainspring about to explode free.

BRRRRRRRRRRRRRRRT!

The snake sent its final warning and I could not react. I could not move. No time to panic. Only an instant to see the white underside of the rattlesnake, to see fangs protruding from a gaping mouth before the rattler landed with a smacking force across my lips.

I tried to lift my arms again, to brush the cold reptile away, but I couldn't move . . . Dammit, I shouted in silence Someone is holding my arms. No, something is holding my arms, and the waves of heat and chills crawled up and down my body as I watched in horror, saw the rattler's head move into my mouth, felt his sharp fangs in my throat.

There was little left for me to do but scream, that God awful silent scream that stayed inside with the snake moving down my throat, into my lungs . . .

"Jay," I could hear Jo's voice calling . . . "Jay, can you hear me?" her voice said getting closer.

I tried to see her. I tried to move, look in the direction of the voice.

"Jay, you are okay," she said, her voice now only a few feet away but I still couldn't see her.

"Jay, the operation was perfect. You are in great shape. Things couldn't be better."

Operation, I thought. What the hell is she talking about. I just went to sleep. They haven't done the operation yet. What's this snake doing in my throat?

"Jay," Jo repeated, "you are all right. Dr. Craver said you went through the operation like a champ. You've had a mammary artery bypass," she said. "They didn't have to take a vein out of your leg. You're doing just great."

Suddenly, I knew where I was. I had been there before. Pinioned like a butterfly with a steel needle through its body. Pinioned; no other word for it. Flat on my back, I am strung with wires, tubes, needles, lines, threads, straps, elastic cords. There is no snake down my throat. Only that God awful tube, but I knew these medical chains, strong and delicate, added up to new life. Power, energy, oxygen, dextrose, liquids dark and light, gases under pressure, drugs to do this and to do that, and I'm back!

But I never left. I was only put to sleep for the operation just minutes ago. That's right, just minutes ago! No, wait! Jo's here . . .

"Jay, can you hear me?" her voice is next to my ear.

I try to answer, but I can't. That damn tube. I nod yes, and strain to see her . . .

"You are fine," she says. "Your operation went perfectly. You got what you wanted," she said. "The mammary artery bypass."

In spite of the tube, in spite of being chained to the bed, I knew where I was and Jo's voice put me at ease. *Here I am* in this thing they call intensive care, and I could hear Jo telling me that the surgery was over. I could hear other people talking, hear the sounds of alarms, bubbling noises. It was over. The operation was complete. It was successful. Time to sleep . . .

"**M**r. Barbree," the voice came through the fog from a distance beyond my present world. "Mr. Barbree," I heard the voice again, "I'm Rebecca, I'm your nurse," the pleasant voice moved closer. "I'm here if you need anything."

I tried to say, thank you, but there was no sound. No words came out, and suddenly I realized that the damn tube was down my throat. I had fought that beast before and therein lay the key. Now was not the time for war but for peace. Do not fight! I told myself. Do not resist. Relax. It was all that was necessary. Relax. Sleep. Relax . . .

*D*r. *John Waller came into CIC (cardiac intensive care), and looked at Rebecca. "How's Jay Barbree doing?" he asked the nurse.*

"He's doing just great," she answered, shaking her head. "Look at the heart rate. Seventy-four, for heaven's sake."

"He went through the surgery the same way," Dr. Waller explained.

"But it should be in the nineties, even in the one hundreds," she protested. "You'd never know he'd just been through open heart surgery."

"His heart was like that before surgery," Dr. Waller smiled. "Strong all the way through. Perfect condition. Too bad most people don't approach heart disease like this."

"Like what?"

"Like taking care of a problem before there's a heart attack, before there's damage," the professor explained. "They come in here looking for magic, looking for us to perform miracles after they've done all the wrong things, after luck has smiled on them and they've survived a heart attack."

The nurse nodded in agreement.

"If they would just practice prevention . . . ," the professor said, his voice trailing away.

The nurse nodded again in agreement.

"Well, most don't," Dr. Waller said, moving to check out the respirator.

"Think we might take the tube out tonight?" Rebecca asked. *"He's doing so well, and . . ."*

"I'm thinking about it," Dr. Waller interrupted. *"Let's run some tests."*

Voices? *Confusion!*

What's happening? Where am I? How did I get here? What's wrong with me?

I know it's a hospital. That's glaringly obvious from sounds and sights, smells and touch, gleaming equipment, dazzling lights, voices, caring sounds, the sounds of machinery, the *whirr* of fans, heels on the floor, doors opening and closing and—

I'm in bed, I'm tied down in bed. Why am I tied down in bed? I'm connected to these banks of machinery.

Think, Jay, think!

Emory! You're at Emory. The operation.

There. Let me focus on that. On the wall, it's a TV. You know about TV. It's a TV set mounted on the wall. It's in front of your bed. There, it's clear. You can see now.

Cough. Clear your throat. You can't. What the hell is wrong? That tube. It's choking you.

No, no it's not choking me. Relax. It's helping me to breathe. *Good, Lord, I could breathe easier with it out.*

Equipment. Just look at all this equipment.

The tube. It's an endotracheal tube. You know about that, Jay. It goes to the ventilator. It helps you breath during and after surgery. Your lungs. They stopped your lungs when you were cut open. The ventilator makes sure you don't forget to breathe. You know that. You're thinking now. Keep thinking.

All this other stuff. Most of it measures the pressure and function of your heart, checks your blood pressure, follows your heart rate.

"Mr. Barbree," a face appeared before me. "You feel okay?"

I stared. A human. A human among all that equipment. I focused on her eyes and nodded yes.

"You need anything?"

I shook my head no.

"Remember me? I'm Rebecca, your nurse."

I nodded yes.

"It's time to suction your lungs," she said, moving a smaller hose through the inside of my breathing tube. "You may feel like it's gonna' choke you," she added, "but it won't. We'll make it quick."

She was right. I felt the smaller tube move into my lungs and the suction pressure shut down all efforts to breathe. I began to fight it, to twist my body against the restraints holding me to the bed. It was a fight for survival, but instantly it was over, and suddenly I was breathing easier. It was most certainly an improvement.

I relaxed against my bed, my eyes followed her. My mind was clear. I knew where I was and what had happened, and most of all I knew what I must do to recover.

"Here's your call button," Rebecca said, placing my left hand over the device that also contained the button to turn on the TV. The restraints held me at my wrists, but I could move my hands a few inches. I turned on the TV, and began moving it through the channels.

"I don't believe this," the nurse said. "Your gonna' watch television?"

I nodded yes.

"You must be feeling pretty good?"

Again, I nodded yes as I began making writing motions on the sheet with my right hand.

"You want something?"

I nodded yes.

"Write it out for me," Rebecca smiled.

My index finger moved across the sheet spelling the word *wife*.

"You want your wife?"

I nodded yes.

"She's outside. She'll be able to come in during visiting hours," Rebecca said. "That won't be too long from now."

Jo sat in the waiting room, lying on a long couch, claiming squatters rights for what she knew would be a long night.

"You're not gonna' sleep on that couch are you?" an elderly gentleman stood before her. "That's my couch," he said firmly.

"Oh, okay," Jo replied without threat. She didn't want a confrontation.

"My wife has been here for two weeks," the elderly gentleman continued. "I've been sleeping on that couch every night."

"That's fine," Jo smiled, getting up, "the couch is yours."

"You sleep on that one over there," he said, pointing to a shorter bench.

Jo moved to the other couch and placed her pillow and blanket on the end. "I guess we'll be able to go in soon."

The elderly gentleman nodded.

"Your wife have open heart surgery?"

He nodded again.

"How's she doing?"

"Not too well," he replied. "They've been trying to get her straightened out. She can't breathe without that machine."

"Really?"

"They'll get her straightened out," he said confidently. "They're the best here."

Jo nodded in agreement.

"You snore?"

Jo was startled by the sudden question. "Not that I know of," she smiled.

"I do," he said. "If I get to snoring too loud tonight, you just shake me."

"I'll do that," Jo smiled.

"Mr. Barbree," Rebecca said, "Dr. Waller is checking the possibility that we may be able to take this tube out tonight."

I nodded, delighted with the idea, as I continued to drift in and out of sleep, occasionally aware that Rebecca was there checking on my breathing, taking measurements to see if the tube could be removed.

Jo came in during visiting hours and she brought me up-to-date on family members, the success of the operation, how well things were going in general.

Later, Rebecca and Dr. Waller adjusted my breathing tube and decided to leave it in during the night. The professor reasoned I was too sleepy for him to guarantee that I would be safe without being connected to the respirator.

I went back to sleep disappointed, but at least I slept. I would later learn Jo stayed at her post in the waiting room most of the night, fighting the sounds of snoring, and when dawn came it was a welcome relief for her. She didn't have the heart to wake the elderly gentleman to complain. After all, he had been there two weeks, standing by for his wife if he should be needed.

The first waking moments for me the day after my surgery came with the removal of the tube from my throat. I spent several minutes gulping in air, breathing heavily and deeply, enjoying the freedom of using my lungs the way nature intended.

I felt great. Enjoyed watching the TODAY SHOW, and assured the nurses that I wasn't in pain. They seemed confused that I was so comfortable, so glad to be alive, so appreciative.

I had long felt that Americans are the biggest cry-babies in the world. For years we in the broadcast profession have drummed into people that any twinge of pain is to be dashed with a pill. It is something not to be tolerated, and if we should sense the slightest hint of it, we should panic.

The truth is, despite our knowledge of pain medications, we know very little about pain, about what causes it, how to deal with it.

Most important of what we don't know is that most pain is self-inflicted, that it is not always an indication of an illness. It is the result, some times, of inadequate exercise, of a poor diet, insufficient sleep, overeating, excessive drinking, and all too often comes from stress, worry, tension, boredom and sometimes, suppressed rage.

The simplest and best way to eliminate pain is to rid your body of the cause. Don't immediately reach for painkillers. Learn to live with a mild degree of discomfort. That way, you will have a true picture of how you really feel.

I shifted my body and continued to enjoy my newly reacquainted ability to breathe freely. Wow! It was great to be rid of that breathing tube, and I knew the cause of any pain I felt the morning after my operation was obvious. My body had been cut open by an air-driven saw—the two halves of my chest had been spread apart, and the heart had been handled and repaired. And while this was going on, the heart and lungs had been stopped to make the job easier.

Yep, I knew why I felt some discomfort, but it was more important to me to retain my sense of feel, to be alert, to understand what was happening instead of recovering in an unfeeling fog for several days.

That afternoon, less than a day after I had left surgery, I was moved into a room where I would spend a week being monitored while I gained strength.

I sensed that Jo was even happier than I about my being moved out of Intensive Care. She had endured the discomfort of trying to sleep on that short couch in the waiting room. The sight of a rollaway bed and a bathroom equipped with a shower, brought a broad smile to her face. Watching her I reminded myself that some people were not as lucky as I was to have such a partner for life.

We both knew the worst was over and that time was now my friend. I would simply lie there and rest, follow doctor's orders, and help my body heal.

My doctor, Dr. Spencer King III, dropped by to see me and took me off most of my medication. He kept me on my beta blocker Inderal (once on the drug it is dangerous to stop as I learned when my brother died. Withdrawal must be gradual with the dosage being stair-stepped down over a period of time), and he maintained my dosage of Quinidine

Sulfate (an old, dependable drug that has proven itself as an agent that keeps the heart happy, keeps it beating regularly).

Even though Professor King is one of the country's foremost doctors, I had long ago promised my own doctor, Onkar Narula, that I would not permit anyone to change my medication without his consent. I owed him a phone call to report on the operation, and, of course, he was pleased that everything had gone so well. He was also in perfect agreement with Dr. King's appraisal of my medication needs. He explained that the most important drug for me at the moment was the Quinidine Sulfate because my heart had just been stopped, handled, and restarted, and for the next five days it should be kept quiet and treated most gently.

Well, the old heart astonished them all by never missing a beat, and after a week and a couple of visits by Dr. Joseph Craver who explained my surgery completely, I was ready to leave the hospital.

I had been fully instructed on how I should spend the next four to six weeks recovering at home. The most disappointing order was for me not to drive. The doctors were concerned that I not be involved in an accident. A slam into the steering wheel could break my chest open before the bones had time to mend. This made perfect sense to me, but I didn't have to like it.

We loaded up the car, and with me as co-pilot, Jo drove us through the streets of east Atlanta until we found the bypass that took us to Interstate 75. There was something good, relaxing, and reassuring about the freedom of the open road, and we happily motored through the heart of Georgia to the Florida line.

There, we pulled into the Holiday Inn where we had spent the night on our way to Atlanta. We both had promised ourselves to return and we felt good. In fact, we felt blessed. We had, thanks to the Almighty, been given another chapter in our lives together, possibly even another book.

All smiles, we relaxed under the pines, in the peaceful, out-of-the-way retreat.

We spent the following day driving home, where our first stop was to see how the construction on our house was coming along. Our builder and friend, Henry Goolsby, had the crews whipped into shape and we loved what we saw. But more important, I was happy that I was alive to see it, to have the opportunity to live in our dream house.

We drove on to the condo we were renting, and when we went through the door my eyes suddenly filled with tears. Balloons and streamers and welcome home signs greeted me. My daughters, grandson, and friends had used computers to print out huge signs reading, "Welcome home, Dad!"—"We love You!"—each of them bordered with hearts and appropriate drawings.

I stood there crying, happy tears falling down my face.

TWENTY-FIVE

"All Creatures Small And Large"

The New York director's voice came through the IFB (interrupted feedback) line into my ear piece. *"You're at the top of the show, Jay. We'll be coming to you in eight minutes."*

"Thank you," I acknowledged. "We're ready."

"You hear that okay, Jay?" Dale Hancock, the studio engineer asked.

"Yeah, fine Dale."

With the coming of spring, Jo and I had moved into our new home on the lake and NBC-TV had increased my responsibilities. I was given the assignment of covering Mission Control in Houston during the space shuttle flights as well as covering the Cape Canaveral launch site.

The new assignment pleased me greatly.

I had made a problem-free recovery from my bypass operation and each day was a new adventure. I was living life with gratitude for every hour and being back in Houston, doing the television reports, took me back to the days of the Gemini missions and the Apollo moon landings, made me feel young again, sent me back to my youth.

Rod Prince, the domestic assignment editor in New York had said, "Jay, you know more about space than anyone. I want you to cover the mission from liftoff to landing."

"I'll be happy to, Rod."

"Science editor Bob Bazell will cover most of the highlights, but you'll be the general space correspondent."

"Thank you, Rod," I said simply, knowing Prince had no idea what his actions had done for my self esteem, for my dignity.

I had much to be thankful for and I began my new life and assignment with a simple promise to do the best I possibly could.

"Jay, six minutes," the director's voice came through my ear piece.

"Jay, this is Jamie Gangel, can you hear me?"

"Loud and clear, Jamie."

"You'll be at the top of show."

"Thank you, Jamie."

It was difficult to express how good I felt about myself. How the recovery from the operation, the knowing that my heart was receiving the blood it needed, made me feel about life. Hostility was no longer a dominant force in my attitude. It had been replaced with appreciation.

I seemed to have rediscovered something I had learned a long time ago, a kindness and gentleness my sister Billie and I had discovered in the woods of Kentucky. I was twelve, she was fourteen, and we thought we would go hunting.

We took the family's smallest shotgun, a .20 gauge, and went into the woods. It was spring, the trees were fresh with green. Life rushed about, squirrels running and leaping from limb to limb, playing and searching for food.

I took aim, pulled the trigger, and a young squirrel fell to the ground. We quickly ran over to collect our game. But what we found was not a dead animal for cooking, but a live, wounded creature, fighting for life.

Billie and I gathered the young squirrel in our arms, took him home and nursed him back to health. He returned to the woods, and we returned the shotgun to its rack. If eating meat meant we had to kill the creature, we would go without. Vegetables would do us nicely.

"Jay, four minutes."

I glanced at the clock and network monitor mounted on the desk before me. The red second hand slipped through the vertical. Dale Hancock stood behind the camera. Bureau Coordinator Joyce Barnell, who could locate a pigmy's gonad if you needed one, was on the phone, making sure nothing came unglued. Producer Ray Elberfeld kept updating editorial content while engineers Sally Benson and Rick Rodriguez kept the equipment working. Barbara Joy monitored mission control.

I grinned. We couldn't be more ready.

I had been in Houston four days covering the mission and things could not have gone better. We had delivered on every request of the network shows and had fulfill the wishes of our affiliates with live reports with their anchors. We had done all this without one single unkind word among us. Amazing, I thought.

"This is the fourth day, and by now we should have had at least two fights," Producer Ray Elberfeld had said earlier.

"You won't get a fight with me," I smiled. "Not anymore, if I can help it."

Ray nodded. "I've really enjoyed working with you, Jay."

"Thank's, Ray. You're a good producer. It's easy working with people who know what they're doing."

I was pleased, but more than that, grateful, for my performance. I really felt like the recovering alcoholic. I was getting over lifelong hostility and I knew I had to take it one day at a time.

Keeping on my health self-management program was no big deal. It was a chosen lifestyle, as routine as putting your favorite clothes on, brushing your teeth. But getting control of your attitude, changing inherited hostility is a tall order.

However, I was determined to do just that. And I did. Even the typical everyday arguments between husband and wife were coming with less frequency between Jo and me.

After screaming no, no, no, many times, Jo even gave in and let me plant my coconut palms in a suitable spot in the yard. It was difficult for her to understand what the fragile trees meant to me. How important it was for us to nurse them back to health after the December freeze, but as always she wanted me to be happy and trusted me to tell her how.

"One minute, Jay."

I sat up straight. Checked my tie and took a final glance at my notes. I wouldn't be reading anything. It was important to adlib live openings and closings, and respond to questions with the same realism. To be natural was the key.

"Forty-five seconds, Jay."

I cleared my throat, the final reflex action before facing the live television camera.

Through my earpiece I could hear Jamie Gangel opening the show in New York, voicing the billboard.

"Thirty seconds, Jay."

I studied Dale Hancock behind the camera, right hand poised above his head, waiting to throw the cue.

Through my earpiece I heard Jamie introduce our report: *"Discovery is in high earth orbit as its four-man, one-woman crew prepares to deploy the Hubble Space Telescope.*

"The telescope is considered one of the most important scientific payloads ever built, and at $1.5 billion, it's the most expensive.

"We get the latest on the mission from NBC's Jay Barbree who is at the Johnson Space Center.

"Good morning, Jay."

Studio engineer Dale Hancock brought his hand down. In my earpiece a single word: *"go!"*

"Good morning, Jamie.

"Discovery's astronauts were awakened for their most important day in space by a personalized song written by their training team and a local band," I said slowly and clearly.

The studio shot of me on the monitor switched to a shot of Discovery high above the earth. From the television speakers a song:

> *"Good morning outer space*
> *"From all the human race*
> *"It's time to stow your sleeping gear . . ."*

The report continued for another minute and was one of ten live television feeds I made during the Hubble Space Telescope mission. I never lost my temper. I was proud of myself.

As I thought about it I knew the weeks I spent recovering from my bypass operation were successful, I had reprogrammed my attitude to bring me to this point.

It was obvious that during the year which had preceeded the bypass my self-management health program had contributed to keeping my coronary artery disease within control, but it was also obvious, and how I hated to admit it, that there was failure.

The number one cause of the failure was, of course, heredity, but hostility, cynical mistrust, perfectionism, and intolerance for others were equal contributors.

I spoke with Dr. Gerald Fletcher, Professor of Cardiology and Chairman of the Rehabilitation Center at the Emory University School of Medicine, and the first thing he told me was, "Jay, don't solely blame yourself for your coronary artery disease. Blame the genes you inherited."

"I'm beginning to understand that," I replied.

"The lesions most likely started in your coronary arteries when you were only seven or eight years old," he added, "and all your efforts in fighting the disease succeeded in slowing down the growth. That's what makes your prevention program worthwhile."

I had long understood the need for such a prevention program, and I also knew my self-help efforts were the direct reason that had brought me from the PETscan test to the mammary artery bypass operation that prevented any damage to my heart.

I also knew I was a good example of how a change in life style, drugs, and surgery is pushing death by heart disease further into old age.

The progress against coronary disease between 1968 and 1988 surprised even the most optimistic observers. The death rate by heart disease plunged forty-eight percent during the two decades, not only because of a revolution in surgery, angioplasty, and drugs, but because of a healthier national life style.

For example, researchers say Americans drink half the high-saturated-fat whole milk they did in the 1960s, eat far less red meat, ingest little cholesterol, and consume far less fat in general.

The same researchers tell us if Americans will also exercise more, the coronary heart disease death rate will plummet further in the 1990s.

Specialists are finding more dependable ways (the PET-scan for example) to detect the disease early. New drugs and treatment strategies promise to prevent, or even to reverse, the plaque forming lesions in the coronaries.

For the '90s and beyond, scientists have developed miniature ultrasound probes that will be inserted into the body to take 3-D pictures of the heart's arteries. The pictures will clearly show cracks and breaks in the artery wall, bulges of fatty deposits and the layers of tissue that surround the blood vessel.

On a television screen, doctors will be able to look down the artery, examine the muscle that surrounds it or even open it up and explore the rough, snaking surface that blood flows over.

They will be able to rotate the pictures side to side, or end to end to give them the best perspective on the contours they need to smooth away or work around.

The new high-resolution pictures will permit doctors to determine whether the clogged arteries require bypass surgery or if the blockage can be opened with balloon angioplasty.

If angioplasty is chosen, the pictures will also allow doctors to see if it was successful and if the artery will remain open, and if cholesterol-lowering drugs are reducing the buildup of fatty deposits.

With the new equipment and techniques being developed, by the time a Baby Boomer retires at sixty-five, about the year 2011, heart disease should no longer rob most people of a normal life span.

Dr. William Castelli, the director of the famed Framingham Heart Study group, predicts that if the trend toward lower cholesterol continues, we could have another dramatic fall in coronary death rates in the next decade.

"We'll look back and see heart disease as unique to the Twentieth Century," says Edward Schneider, a gerontologist with the University of Southern California.

There's good reason to believe these predictions will

come true because life expectancy for Americans has risen five years (to about seventy-five years of age) since the 1960s because of the progress made against heart disease. Four hundred twenty thousand Americans alive today would have died in 1989 alone had the coronary heart disease death rate not dropped.

Doctors have gotten to this point largely by whittling away at the three chief coronary heart disease risk factors— smoking, high blood pressure and high cholesterol.

Statisticians report lowering the coronary risk factors accounted for two-thirds of the lives saved between 1968 and 1976, and the risks are being cut even more. Smoking rates among some groups (those under twenty and blue collar workers) are still high but continue to drop. Less than a third of American males smoke, compared with a majority in the 1960s. Low-fat foods are also lowering the risks.

Winning the battle will be mainly a matter of preventive medicine. The disease can be arrested in two-thirds of those who already have damaged arteries which includes most American men by age forty.

What I needed protection from could not yet be offered —a defense against inherited heart disease and an inherited hostile attitude.

Researchers are daily becoming aware how important such risk factors as stress and hostility are. As said earlier, studies have suggested that hard-driving "type A" people, especially those displaying hostility, are more likely to develop coronary artery disease than calmer people.

Scientists in studies using monkeys made half the animals in an experiment anxious by moving them frequently from cage to cage, from one monkey group to another. A control group ate the same diet, a typical one with fat, but these animals weren't on the move. Like hostile types on the run, the monkeys under stress were constantly struggling to dominate their changing peer groups.

These animals developed more atherosclerosis, and the monkeys whose pulses quickened more than average during stress, the so-called high reactors, developed twice the coronary artery damage.

Scientists now believe that certain human beings are

also high reactors, a trait that can easily be checked, and that is an important risk factor for heart disease.

For me, the fight against hostility has already begun, and I am doing everything I can to stay out of situations that breed hostility. Staying out of heavy, bumper-to-bumper traffic, and constantly reminding myself to mellow out, to be more trustful and tolerant of others. Now I refuse to permit fellow workers to goad me into crisis situations. My work is getting done, I am still out in front with my coverage of the space program, and I find myself getting the news out in a more relaxed manner.

In regards to heredity, I see researchers already closing in on isolating the genes that predispose people like myself to heart disease. Genetic tests may disclose defects in cholesterol metabolism that contribute to atherosclerosis, and may lead to new ways, including drugs, to deal with the clogging of coronary arteries caused by heredity.

But the flip side to heredity and hostility drawbacks is peace and laughter, and I find myself searching for quiet, restful, private places more often—places where I can think of something funny, where I can laugh and enjoy life.

There is evidence the human body is programmed to start its own steady walk toward death from the moment a person is born, and man spends much of his life trying to strike down the diseases that are gradually sapping the life out of him.

Have you ever noticed how some people in their sixties, seventies, and eighties walk around with a perpetual frown on their faces. They never seem to be happy. Their hostility and cynical mistrust is killing them.

Studies suggest that one of the best weapons against dying is having someone to grow old with, to share your final years with, to share happy memories and daily accomplishments with as you near the end of your time on earth.

Most people are convinced they would like to live forever, to find a cure for death itself. But, when you think about this, do you really think most people could tolerate endless life? I think not. Forever is such a long time.

But while here living life to its fullest and with meaning, and most importantly, with happiness and laughter, is the answer. And when this quality of life can not be maintained, then it is time to move on, to the other side.

Since my bypass operation I am beginning to understand this, and in talking with other fellow bypassers, members of what we call "The Zipper Club" because of the long incision down our chests, I find that they too have come to similar conclusions.

I am blessed with a wonderful wife, a good job, with top-notch bosses, and the move into my new home has brought me to the quiet lake, to the peaceful neighborhood of which I always dreamed. I have brought myself to the state of mind wherein I can enjoy it.

T WENTY-SIX

"That's A Wrap"

A weather front had passed over northern Florida and left behind a sky of rare clarity. There were the whitest of puffy clouds floating against a rich, clean blue, and beneath this portrait of a perfect day were stands of pine lost in a mass of green. A murky landscape, heavily thatched with moss hanging from oaks, spreads of algae, tall grass verdant in the rain-rich spring.

I drove at a steady pace, my car followed by sun reflections leaping along the surface of cypress ponds, moss-hung growth on each side of the concrete ribbon slashing through the piney forests—Interstate 95 running north and south.

The landscape unfolded familiar secrets to me. I had first driven the same land in another spring long ago when I moved to Cape Canaveral where I would meet my wife Jo, raise a family, and build a life; where I would be hired by NBC News and spend a life covering the space program—a life that has had its contract renewed on this morning of this new perfect day.

I was returning from Jacksonville where my third PET-scan exam had confirmed that the talents of Dr. Joe Craver and the Emory staff had restored full blood flow to my entire heart.

I remembered what Dr. Donald Gordon had said, "It's the most dramatic change I have ever seen following a by-pass operation."

"Just perfect, just perfect," said Dr. David Hess, pointing at the bright reds indicating blood flow in the series of pictures that were made by the computer.

The smiling physicians and their staff agreed that the results of my mammary artery bypass operation were the best they had ever seen, and there was a lot of back-slapping, faces supporting wide grins. Good results had been expected, but not the dramatic blood flow improvement recorded by the PETscan. Every fiber of my heart was now receiving blood, and it was the confirmation needed to put my mind at ease.

When they told me they didn't want to see me for three or four years, my grin was the largest.

The drive home from Jacksonville gave me time to think, to reflect, to be alone with my thoughts.

Foremost in my mind was the peaceful knowledge that my mammary artery bypass operation had been such a success and with it came the promise of more life.

I drove home grinning.

Because of the talents of Dr. Joe Craver and the Emory staff, I felt it was a time of renewal of life, and as I neared my house, I could see the same weather front that had cleaned the skies the night before with its heavy rains had brought trees and lawns and gardens surging to life. Azalea and bougainvillea and oleander blossoms painted a never-ending picture of the change of seasons along the streets I traveled, and in the distance was the darker coloring of the banks along the Banana River.

I drove down Tropical Trail on Merritt Island and when I reached our street, I turned into the drive which winds down to the curving shore of Honeymoon Lake. Our new home, sitting on a hill facing the water, appeared suddenly, and I drove into the circular drive that weaves its way through the live oaks standing sentry about the house.

Jo stood in the oriental sunken garden, a water hose in her hands, and I stopped the car.

"How did it go?" she asked.

"Better than expected," I smiled. "Dr. Craver and his gang did their jobs exceptionally well," I added, launching into a full report on the PETscan exam.

When I finished, Jo grinned and said, "I guess you're gonna' live?"

"Yep, you're stuck."

She nodded, a soft smile of relief crossed her lips.

I stood in the drive looking down at her. She was dressed in an old shirt, in shorts, her face moist with sweat from tending the garden, but never had she been more radiant. She was beautiful in a way I'd never known before.

It had been three years since I dropped dead jogging, and between self-help, faith, and medical help, we both had changed. Life was different, every second full of new meaning.

I had a sudden urge. "Let's drive to the beach," I said.

"Right now?"

"Right now!"

"Okay," she said, recognizing before I did what was in my mind. I wanted to go to the spot, the place where I fell, and celebrate my victory of sorts over death. I suppose that wasn't too hard to understand but it wasn't all of that big of a deal.

We put the top down and drove out of our driveway, around the lake, and soon we were on the causeway, headed for the ocean. We both enjoyed the spring air rushing past our face, through our hair. It seemed I had forgotten just how blue the Florida sky could be.

It was a perfect day in so many ways and the visit to the beach seemed especially appropriate. We parked at Second Street and walked the crossover to the bottom of the stairs where we quickly rid ourselves of our shoes.

We walked up the beach, behind our old house, with the wind to our backs. It caught the loose strands of Jo's hair and blew them about her face. We walked with our shoulders touching, she clasping my arm tight, and silently we crossed the sand where I had fallen and stood there a few moments.

There was nothing to say. It had all been said. We both knew what lay behind and what lay ahead.

Suddenly we stopped, turned around and stared at where we had been. "Our footprints, Jay," Jo said smiling. "Look at them. They belong together."